FUKUSHIMA MELTDOWN AND MODERN RADIATION:

PROTECTING OURSELVES AND OUR FUTURE GENERATIONS

JOHN W. APSLEY II, MD(E), ND, DC

Temet Nosce Publications

Published in the United States by:

Temet Nosce Publications
Sammamish, WA 98075
www.DoctorApsley.com

Library of Congress Cataloging-in-Publication Data:

Fukushima meltdown and modern radiation: protecting ourselves and our future generations: radiation, regeneration, cellular health, nuclear power / by John W. Apsley II

Includes bibliographic references and works.

ISBN 978-0-945704-07-2

Dedication

I dedicate this book to:

Maggie and Arnie Gundersen
and their continuing crusade to
protect the world from nuclear fallout.

My family, their children and their
children's children down though
the course of time.

Acknowledgements

I have attempted to give a clear and understandable summary of radiation toxicity as it truly is and will be for centuries to come.

This work would not have been possible without the invaluable contributions of several people to whom I will always be most grateful.

Arnie and Maggie Gundersen of www.fairewinds.com, guided me through much of the overwhelming real-time data pouring endlessly out of the Fukushima Catastrophe. They helped insure the data was accurately described and placed into proper context. Their contributions have all been truly brilliant and most generous.

My wife, Linda, meticulously edited, formatted and programmed the final manuscript so that it could become highly readable and available in all forms currently offered by the digital age. This book would never have reached completion without her many years of literary prowess and publishing expertise.

What comes repeatedly to my mind are the words of Albert Einstein when he stated, "A foolish faith in authority is the worst enemy of truth" (letter to a friend, 1901).

Many thanks to the three other Nobel Laureates, including Linus Pauling, Andrei Sakharov and Helen Caldicott, founding member of the Nuclear Policy Research Institute or NPRI (www.nuclearpolicy.org).

Special appreciation to Abram Petkau and the decades long work of the Radiation Public Health Project (http://www.radiation.org).

I would also like to acknowledge the monumental work of and achievements of Alexey V. Yablokov et al., for their book: *Chernobyl: Consequences of the Catastrophe for People and the Environment*, as well as to Chris Busby, Scientific Secretary to the European Committee on Radiation Risk (www.euradcom.org).

I would also like to make special mention to both the Union of Concerned Scientists (http://www.ucsusa.org) as well as Greenpeace (http://www.greenpeace.org/usa/en/) for their relentless pursuit of the truth in as far as the limitations, liabilities, political intrigue and economic realities of nuclear power generation are concerned.

My work has benefitted from Mark Starr's, MD, tireless efforts to properly explain the role our most vital Thyroid gland plays in our constitutional health, from cradle to grave. His work captured in *Hypothyroidism Type 2*, more than any other book I am aware of provides the best light on proper thyroid medication dosage so all may heartily avoid the grave before their time.

These exceptional researchers and organizations have spent much time, energy and focus selflessly alerting the general public not only to the dangers of splitting the atom no matter to what purpose, but also to the nature of the political beast that relentlessly pursues its exploitation, no matter what the cost.

Contents

Preface

As I wrote this book *Fukushima Meltdown & Modern Radiation: Protecting Ourselves and Our Future Generations,* I kept reminding myself of the words spoken by Albert Einstein who stated, "Nuclear power is one hell of a way to boil water."[1] Now I understand what he meant – it is clearly a technology straight from hell. Nuclear power has brought unprecedented and ever compounding damage into our global environment. The current and past impact of nuclear radioactive releases alone will negatively impact generations for hundreds if not thousands of years. We would be wise to follow the lead of both Germany and Italy to shift expeditiously from nuclear power to safer and less expensive technologies.[2] When taking the facts as a whole and using common sense with no spin attached, the most expensive, dangerous and geopolitically riskiest means to generate electricity is from nuclear power.[3, 4, 5, 6, 7]

As a researcher and clinical specialist in regeneration, I have a unique understanding of how humans may regenerate their cellular structure and functions. Evidence from cultures thriving in the "Blue-Zones" across the world (where the locals live essentially disease free and do not begin their aging process until decades after an average American starts theirs), suggests that health for most of people in the world is heading in the wrong direction.[8]

When I published my second book on human regeneration in 1996, I ran across a series of startling articles concerning man-created releases of radioactive fallout that now permeate the globe. It was apparent to me then that there is a clear cause and effect relationship between global radioactive fallout and the rise in chronic degenerative diseases. In America, in the decades immediately prior to the nuclear age, the rate of chronic degenerative disease was declining. And as soon as mankind gave birth to the nuclear age, chronic degenerative diseases started climbing at an alarming pace with no relief in sight.[9]

As of 2011, science reveals the many facets of the aging process; first and foremost is free-radical pathology. People who live long lives are able to minimize their exposure to toxic free radicals as well as efficiently quench cell damage caused by free-radicals. Free-radicals are essentially rogue electron infernos that burn and char our tissues at the cell and below cell levels. Like a miniaturized raging forest fire, free-radicals accelerate our aging process 24/7. A good example would be if you poured hydrogen peroxide directly onto a fresh scrape. It burns like hell for a few seconds, doesn't it?

Long-lived cultures have mastered a lifestyle that surrounds, contains and neutralizes free radicals using four strategies I term the Four Pillars of Regeneration. All these cultures have passed down efficient means to detoxify their bodies of toxins, and their universal fitness harnesses the power of oxygen to lessen the production of free-radicals. At the same time, their daily diet includes potent neutralizers to any free-radical that might arise, and finally, their environment and culture produces a profound sense of spiritual gratitude and harmony that removes additional internal stress.

It is clear to me that we are degenerating as a race, and not thriving as many in modern conventional medicine would like us to believe. Unfortunately, our modern culture has left behind these four pillars to longevity and extreme health in favor of stress and the generation of more stress, and those stresses often translate into free-radical pathology.

I decided to write this book mainly because I have three grandkids now plus a fourth one on the way. I have spent my adult life protecting the health of my family and sharing my knowledge with anyone who has ears to hear. My grandchildren are entering a time when it will be more difficult to protect health. As the challenges become greater, the opportunities for our awareness become keener. My hope is that awareness of the need to act will span the globe and encourage people to develop new health practices.

My goal in writing *Fukushima Meltdown & Modern Radiation* now is to give you tools to help yourself and your family overcome the effects of global radioactivity. *Fukushima Meltdown & Modern Radiation* is a combination of my knowledge of cellular regeneration combined with my significant research into the subject of radioactivity, especially the poisons emitted through radioactive fallout. Finally, *Fukushima Meltdown & Modern Radiation* gives you the reader antidotes for good health and easy-to-use recipes to help your body defend itself against the constant onslaught of new environmental toxins.

For your reading ease, I have divided this book into three parts. In Part I, I explain the current state of radioactivity in our global environment, with a focus on Japan and the United States. In Part II, I document lifestyle changes you can implement to protect your health. Finally, in Part III, I explain how to change your diet to accomplish comprehensive protection.

I have structured the book to give you the tools to protect your family:

- ✓ First, become properly informed about the crises of radiation and pass the information along to as many folks as possible.
- ✓ Second, facilitate elimination of any prior internal contamination.

- ✓ Third, augment repair of prior damage from contamination.
- ✓ Fourth, prevent or minimize new exposure to insidious bioaccumulations of radioactive particles, or all other sources of radiation.
- ✓ Fifth, keep antioxidant repair systems at healthy levels to quickly handle any new exposures that slip through.
- ✓ Sixth, help prevent trans-generational transference down your family's tree.

We already have a significant backlog of damage, so fixing that damage will require careful planning. I recommend starting by first protecting yourselves and your loved ones, while preserving your strength to help your community and the society at large. After mastering and implementing the various techniques in this book, you should turn your energy and resources toward the prevention of future catastrophes involving radioactive materials. By working together, we can cut the snake's head off by quickly developing power generating technologies that will make nuclear power obsolete, and thereby protect our immediate future generations from radiation.

We must make our voices heard throughout our political system, as has recently occurred both in Germany and in Italy. Japan has just recently opened up to the idea that just one nuclear power plant catastrophe costs more economically than the total accumulated profits from their entire fleet of nuclear power electrical generating plants.

Finally, it is my utmost wish that we may all unite to change our lives for the better. We must work together to find the means to change the manner in which we live closer to that of the long-living cultures that still may be found around the world. We must work together to benefit from modern technology that is in harmony with Nature, and that means we must immediately implement easier, simpler and cheaper means to safely boil water.[10]

Part I

No Singing in the Black Rain

Nuclear power generation is the most dangerous means to produce electricity due to its production of radioactive particles which retain destructive ionizing power for hundreds if not thousands of years. Nuclear power plant operation requires the release of small amounts of radiation into the surrounding air and water on a never-ending basis. And the number of nuclear accidents that have gone "under the radar" is larger than most would think (at least 27 world-wide since 1952).[11]

Nuclear power generation is the most expensive means to produce electricity because taxpayers are initially responsible for subsidizing the building of the plant, yet never recoup their investment. These same taxpayers are required to indefinitely subsidize the average monthly costs giving the illusion of lower monthly electrical bills.[12]

Furthermore, the taxpayer financial outlay to decommission obsolete nuclear power plants is an obscene tax burden, yet hardly ever publicized. Plus, consider the endless costs incurred to store the vast amounts of spent nuclear fuel for hundreds of years - all the human security required, all the safe and durable construction requirements, the water and land requirements, etc.[13] And then adding insult to more insult, when the most devastating accidents occur, taxpayers are held fully financially responsible to pay for cleanup and much of the restitution, including medical bills (by way of government sponsored health care reimbursements).[14, 15]

This leads into the massive medical care costs required to treat those sickened by the radioactive poisons. A recent German study of children living near 16 of Germany's nuclear power plants showed dramatic increases in all childhood cancers, especially leukemia.[16] Earlier, an identical trend was detected at 138 nuclear power facilities spanning Great Britain, Canada, Spain, Germany, America and Japan.[17] Children living near these nuclear power facilities incurred significantly higher leukemia rates than kids living away from such facilities. The largest study to date concerning this same trend found that medical costs in locations surrounding 198 nuclear sites and 10 countries are simply staggering and unsustainable. [18, 19]

Last but not least, rogue countries operating nuclear power plants have a continual source of refined radioactive materials technologically easy to convert into weapons of mass destruction. When you consider the huge costs shouldered by taxpayers for keeping homeland security ever-vigilant, and the extreme costs of military intervention when perceived as necessary, can anyone seriously argue that nuclear power generation is a cheap source of abundant electrical energy?

And to those still willing to argue the point, consider the fact that regardless of the radiation source, once it gets into the environment's interconnected ecological systems (better termed biosphere) it becomes a problem for all people on the planet.

Modern man is the victim of the very instrument he values most. Every gain in power, every mastery of natural forces, every scientific addition to knowledge, has proven potentially dangerous, because it has not been accompanied by equal gains in self-understanding and self-discipline.

Lewis Mumford

Chapter One

Radiation and Cellular Health

In August of 1945, St. Francis's Hospital (Uragami Daiichi Hospital) in Nagasaki was located one mile from ground zero. The atomic bomb that exploded killed tens of thousands of Japanese. Many citizens died instantly, and many more passed on within days or weeks of the blast. The Director of Internal Medicine in the hospital, Dr. Tatsuichiro Akizuki, saved all staff members and most hospital patients by having them adhere to a strictly vegetarian diet of uncontaminated brown rice, fermented foods, sea algae and land vegetables. Sweets of all types were strictly forbidden, and salt sufficed as the main condiment. Another hospital exactly one mile from ground zero did not follow this dietary regimen. All other treatments remained constant. The loss of human life due to radiation poisoning suffered at this second nearby hospital approached 100%.[20, 21]

When I first read this story many years ago, I was struck by the profound impact diet can have on health and how much radioactive materials can destroy human life. At the same time, I was struck by the body's ability to heal itself from something as catastrophic as the fallout from a nuclear bomb when consistent steps are taken to promote health and heal damage.

In *Fukushima Meltdown & Modern Radiation: Protecting Ourselves and Our Future Generations,* I will help you understand why every American today is bound to have radioactive particles lodged in their tissues and is continuously exposed to varying types of low-dose radioactive emissions. The need to protect ourselves, our children and our communities from such deadly compounds has never been greater. I will also share with you the potential impact of the Fukushima nuclear disaster on health of people in the United States and throughout the world. In addition, I will begin to teach you how to help your family and friends begin to remove radioactive toxins from the body. Finally, I will help you learn what types of foods and supplements science indicates will help your body begin to heal from the impact of radioactive exposure.

In this chapter, I explain the impact of radiation upon cellular health and provide a brief history of the impact of radiation upon health generally. In addition, I will discuss the scientific studies proving that ongoing low doses of radiation over time can be quite devastating to people's health.

How Radiation Devastates Our Cellular Health

Cellular health is at the core of every person's health. If cells are healthy, the human body is able to fight off disease. If cells are unhealthy, the body suffers a weakened immune system and diseases of different severity. During the past three quarters of a century, the industrial revolution has created thousands of pollutants that threaten cellular health, and hence, the health of our entire civilization.

Ever increasing chemical pollution places downward pressure upon the health of the entire human race as it compromises the very fabric of our human constitution. For example, bioaccumulation of the extremely long lasting radioactive elements magnifies throughout the food chain. This increases rather than decreases the power of radioactive ionization upon all life forms occupying the high-end of the food chain. Plants are at the low end of the food chain. As animals consume contaminated plants, their bodies accumulate more radioactive elements in their tissues. When humans then eat contaminated animal products, they consume the amount stored up in the animal and thereby accumulate more radioactivity. Because human beings live at the top most end of the food chain, unless counter-forces arise, such radioactive bioaccumulation and concentration (i.e., biomagnification) disrupts our immunity, longevity and reproductive cycles with mutating forces for generations.

As the number of chemical compounds in the body increases, the cellular stress increases. At the cellular level, multiple pollutants collecting in the body induce an excessive production of free radicals, which are radicals that rally around "species" of oxygen (radical oxygen species or ROS) or nitrogen (radical nitrogen species or RNS). Both are electron infernos.

When produced and managed in the correct amounts, human beings need select ROS (never RNS though) to ward off microbes that may threaten the health of an organ or tissue. Immune cells are experts in producing and delivering unique ROS to melt down microbes. And to this end, immune cells are specially designed to protect themselves with antioxidants.

Of all the destructive pollutants that have been created by humankind, the radioactive elements (scientifically termed radionuclides) have the most potential to cause serious cell damage. When radionuclides enter the body, they are called internal emitters.[22] They are insidious in their generation of destructive ROS and RNS at the cellular level because they are perennial infernos of silent ionizing energy. Radionuclides such as Iodine-131 (131-I), Cesium-137 (137Cs) and Strontium-90 (90Sr), plus Plutonium-239 (239Pu) and Uranium-238 (238U) are like the "Everlasting Ever Ready" battery of ultimate free radical generators. When these devastating internal emitters are added into the chemical soup attacking our cells, the body has a hard time keeping up with neutralizing the resulting free radicals. By themselves these internal emitters and the free radicals they generate can create enough ROS and RNS to damage health by simply melting and burning cells to death.

Most scientists think in terms of ionizing radiation's impact upon our genes and DNA. Internal emitters easily break the strands of molecules holding the DNA together. Single strand breaks (SSB) and even double strand breaks (DSB) are common when exposed to the melting and burning effects of radionuclide ROS. Fortunately, holistic physicians trained in radioprotective methods are able to significantly prevent and reverse SSB and DSB damage within certain limits,[23] a subject comprehensively covered in detail in Chapters 3, 4 and 7.

Our individual cellular structural integrity is "glued together" in large measure by select lipids and essential phospholipids (i.e., fats, fatty proteins, phosphatidylserine or PS, and phosphatidylcholine or PC).[24] Only recently have scientists recognized the extreme importance ionizing radiation plays in the melting and burning of these essential cellular glues. In terms of lethality, these deleterious effects can easily surpass any simultaneously occurring genetic damage. Fortunately, holistic physicians trained in radioprotective intervention know how to prevent ongoing damage when it arises from internal emitters. This subject is also meticulously covered in Chapters 3, 4, 6 and 7.

Finally, over the past 40 years the world's top cell physiologists have uniquely defined what really operates and governs cell physiology. Damage from internal emitters can be understood at the cell and below cell level only if we have a proper working model to go by. For example, there is highly unique water within cells that operates in an essential alliance with at least four other crucial components.[25] These five components are especially vulnerable to the melting and burning of ionizing radiation, and must be radio protected at all costs. Simultaneously, all accrued damage must also be repaired. With extensive or long-term exposures, nothing less than true cellular regeneration may make the difference between accelerated disability, risks for developing cancer, or even for preventing birth defects in our future children. Fortunately, holistic physicians experienced in radioprotective protocols are able to encourage host tissues to regenerate themselves, a subject painstakingly covered in Chapters 5 and 7.

Radioactive Elements and Chronic Degenerative Diseases

Ionizing radioactive elements serve as the supreme amplifiers to the genesis of all chronic degenerative diseases now plaguing our human civilization. From the onset of exposure and ingestion to even the smallest quantities of radionuclides, the immune system begins to rapidly fail.[26, 27, 28, 29, 30, 31, 32, 33, 34, 35, 36] The impact is especially profound and immediate among the very young, the immune compromised (HIV positive) and the very old. For the first time, Yablokov et al. documented the direct correlation between moderate and low-dose radiation exposure and the most serious neurological conditions. Here are some of the potential outcomes low to high intensity radiation exposure can cause:

- ✓ First symptoms often involve one or more of the following: nausea, headaches, weakness, tongue swelling, tongue soreness, funny metallic taste, loss of smell or taste, eyelashes falling out more frequently and more hair coming out when brushed.
- ✓ Breathing disorders, from bloody noses, frequent colds and coughs, or lung cancer from inhaled radioactive "hot particles" (lots of awareness of this in Japan).
- ✓ Birth defects of varying severity.
- ✓ Neurological disorders develop in the very young and old.
- ✓ More serious blood disorders arise, such as leukemia.
- ✓ Internal organs initiate solid tumor formation, early heart disease, early liver disease and even onset of debilitating muscular-skeletal impairments.
- ✓ Neurological disorders begin to compromise the IQ of offspring and run havoc with depressive mood disorders, and appear to contribute to Autism, suicides and criminal behavior.
- ✓ Chronic degenerative diseases mature and dramatically increase as if a plague has erupted.
- ✓ Neurological disorders concomitantly evolve into Alzheimer's disease, Multiple Sclerosis, Lou Gehrig's disease and Parkinson's disease.

- ✓ Accelerated aging leads more and more frequently to premature death.

Many of the above follow-on injuries have long been observed to occur in children treated with radiation therapy for brain cancer. [37, 38, 39,40, 41, 42] All of the above threaten to undermine every aspect of our modern way of life.[43]

The above conditions result because unless they are checked by interlocking antioxidants, free radicals chew apart the cell from both the outside in, as well as from the inside out. These antioxidants form a highly frail system of checks and balances.[44] This frail checks and balances system quenches free radicals. But this capacity is limited. There are only limited supplies of antioxidants in any given cell, tissue or organ, and those antioxidants must be continually resupplied and/or recharged from dietary sources.[45]

If the ionizing toxins irradiate our cells and tissues and organs 24/7/365, it is essential for our bodies to remove them as quickly as possible, but it doesn't stop there. Once the toxins are removed, our cells and tissues must properly repair the damage (often quite extensive), or risk undergoing a doomed attempt of repair that we define as cancer. Yes, cancer.

Cancer is not just caused by the ionizing radiation directly. Scientific research has determined that cancer results from a doomed attempt of a damaged body to repair itself.[46, 47, 48, 49] How is that? Healthy cellular repair needs all the supporting materials and conditions in the damaged area to be successful. So when the proper supporting elements, signals and cellular environment have been so damaged, deprived or disrupted that healthy repair becomes impossible, the cellular survival program goes rogue, actually making things worse.

Unless we understand radionuclides, learn how they impact our cells and develop a plan for empowering the body to overcome their impacts, we may find our civilization doomed to being cast back into the dark ages of plagues, pestilence, famine and an endless struggle for mere survival. To view this, one needs only travel to the so called inhabitable areas just proximal to the Chernobyl Catastrophe's exclusion zone, such as eastern Belarus.

The recent Fukushima Catastrophe and its potential impact on human health will play out most potently during the next 20 to 30 years. Our challenge is to understand the full potential impact of the atmospheric releases of radioactive materials and to determine what diet and supplement choices will give people the greatest opportunity to maintain good health as we face a brand new and intense attack of free radicals upon our cells. By understanding what is happening in our body and working to make our bodies healthier, each one of us places ourselves and our loved ones in the best possible position to fight the impact of exposure to this radioactivity.

A Brief History of Radiation and its Impact upon Health

Radiation has taken on a whole new meaning since the early dawn of the nuclear age. At first, it was believed that the most dangerous form of radiation poisoning was caused by high doses during a short period of time. However, since the early 1970's, it has been known that long-term exposure to tiny amounts of radiation is much more devastating to the human being.[50] And since 2005, the National Research Council has emphasized that any amount of radiation, no matter how low, is dangerous.[51]

On August 6th, 1945 the United States dropped a 15 Kiloton A-Bomb on Hiroshima, Japan. Then on August 9th, a second 21 Kiloton A-Bomb was dropped on Nagasaki. In both cities combined, either immediately or within the next four months, approximately 200,000 people were killed.[52, 53] These 36 Kilotons of nuclear bombs represent the only nuclear weapons ever detonated in warfare.

Throughout the world, people have mistakenly believed that nuclear power is operated "safely" and only nuclear bombs are dangerous. In fact, the Chernobyl Catastrophe of 1986 was approximately 200 times more powerful than both bombs in terms of the radioactive release.[54] The Chernobyl Catastrophe released 12,000 X 10^{15} Becquerel (Bq) of radioactivity.[55, 56] Using simple division we can determine that the two nuclear bombs dropped on Japan released a total of approximately 60 X 10^{15} Bq of radioactivity compared to Chernobyl's 12,000 x 10^{15} Bq. America's development of nuclear arms at the Hanford nuclear weapons plant located in southeastern Washington State (during and after WWII) released 16,169 X 10^{15} Bq of radioactivity (including ~26 X 10^{15} Bq of radioactive iodine released from 1944 through 1971)[57] into North America's biosphere.[58]

The jet stream carried those radioactive particles in mass to the New York area where they entered the regional biosphere through rainwater (called fallout). Immediately thereafter, New York suffered an unprecedented rise in the number of underweight births. This trend associated with nuclear fallout continued to climb well into the 1960s.[59] The Chernobyl Catastrophe single-handedly released ~3,200 X 10^{15} Bq of 131-I into the atmosphere.[60] In all, over 100 different radionuclides were released. Most were short lived in terms of their toxic radioactivity, but the most dangerous are still present in our global biosphere.[61]

Fallout Spurs Chronic Disease in Our Children

Tragically, up to 212,000 U.S. childhood thyroid cancers would have been avoidable had scientists warned the public to take protective iodine supplementation, and/or thought through their bomb testing methodology.[62] After all, it doesn't take a nuclear scientist to realize that blowing bombs up underground instead of above ground is a better way to avoid spraying our kids with radioactive poisons.

To put in further perspective the damage caused by the nuclear arms radiation, consider the following: Mark Starr, MD, in his outstanding book on *Hypothyroidism Type 2*, explains the long-term implications of health destruction that will result to future generations when the most vital thyroid glands of young Americans become compromised. From 1953 through 1962, tens of millions of Americans were exposed to short-term half-life 131-I, which necessarily destroyed significant amounts of their natural thyroid function for life.[63,64,65,66] Sub-par thyroid function has contributed to catastrophic escalations in all categories of chronic degenerative diseases (i.e., Chronic Fatigue Syndrome, Fibromyalgia, Immune Deficiency syndromes, Cancer, chronic Heart Disease, Diabetes Type II, etc…).[67]

Chart 1.1 reflects the states hardest hit with fallout (especially 131-I) from 1952 through 1963 due to the above ground bomb testing. Folks having children in these areas may have unwittingly set off generational trends reflecting life-long, sub-par thyroid function.

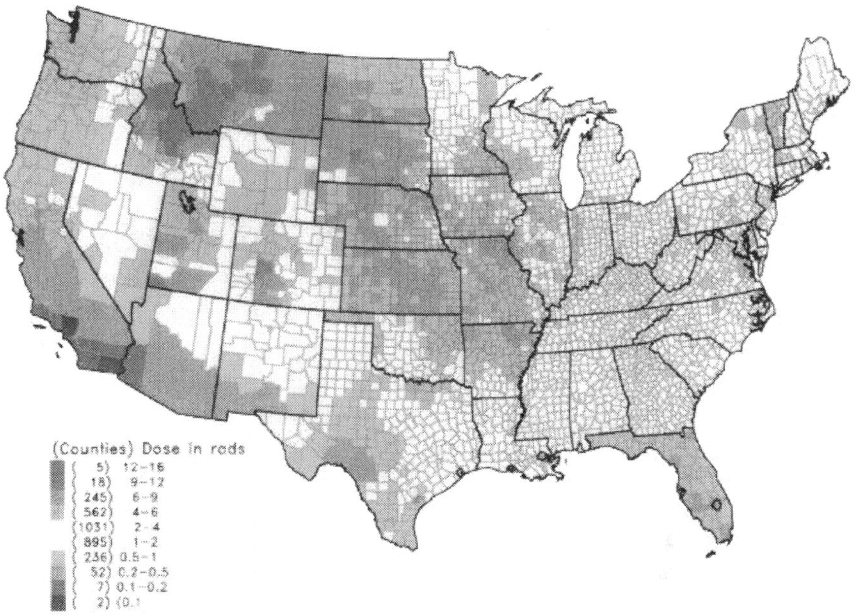

Chart 1.1: Cumulative 1952-1963 Radiation Contamination in America
Source: National Cancer Institute.[68, 69]

Debilitating and destructive longer half-life radionuclides from atmospheric bomb testing are still present in the global biosphere and will continue to be a major catalyst inducing chronic diseases for many generations to come.[70]

From 1953 through 1962, above ground detonation of 541 nuclear bombs yielding altogether 440,000 Kilotons (440 Megatons) was carried out across the globe. The fallout from these above ground nuclear detonations rose to +1,000,000 X 10^{15} Bq.,[71] or hundreds of times more radioactivity than the Chernobyl Catastrophe.[72] The total release of 137Cs into the biosphere from these 541 nuclear bombs has been estimated to be 912 X 10^{15} Bq compared to 280 X 10^{15} Bq arising from the Chernobyl Catastrophe. [73]

Presently, no fewer than 400 million people inhabit areas contaminated by Chernobyl.[74] Outside of Europe, no less than 150 million people were contaminated with Chernobyl's fallout. Recorded debilitating injuries in the regions surrounding Chernobyl have affected eight million people. Less than 1% of North America was contaminated with approximately 1% of the total Chernobyl fallout.[75] In other words, North America got off easy compared to the regions adjoining Chernobyl - eastern Belarus, north central Ukraine and southwestern Russia. In the coming pages, the total number of those who suffered from the Chernobyl Catastrophe will be enumerated, including folks living in North America.

During the past two decades, there has been a sharp increase in underweight births in the Ukraine linked to the Chernobyl Catastrophe. And as of 2007, scientists discovered that only 20% of the children living and growing up in the greater Chernobyl regions were healthy! Prior to the Chernobyl Catastrophe, up to 90% of the children growing up in these same regions were known to be healthy.[76]

As far back as 1993, Sanderson reported that examinations on 30,000 Russian children revealed all had been exposed with up to 100 Ci/km^2 (3.7×10^6 Bq/m^2) of radiation.[77] With such high levels of deadly exposure, it is no wonder that children have suffered so greatly! At that time, this exposure resulted in 70% of the children having abnormal blood pressure, 66% having abnormal thyroid function, 39% having abnormal eye function, 44% having swollen lymph nodes, 35% of boys suffering complete arrest of sexual maturation, and 100% suffering from 100 times what ought to be the normal radiation excreted in their urine. The overall number of Russian children at risk approximated 5,000,000.

As of 1993, 14 million people were living in the potentially lethal fallout zone of Chernobyl's aftermath. The death toll was reportedly so high that attempts were made at the highest official levels to minimize reporting the numbers.[78]

Unfortunately for us, in terms of just 137Cs released, data collected from the worldwide network of the Comprehensive Nuclear-Test-Ban Treaty Organization (CTBTO) in Vienna suggests that the Fukushima Catastrophe equaled one entire Chernobyl Catastrophe as of March 17th, 2011.[79] This suggests that by March 17th, 280 X 10^{15} Bq of 137Cs had already been volatilized into the greater environment.[80] So how many more multiples of Chernobyl's total release of 137Cs may we expect from the ongoing Fukushima Catastrophe?

As of July 2011, 137Cs as well as a host of other radionuclides kept escaping into the ground water, into the ocean and into the air where they were carried into the jet stream and eventually fell across the globe in rain water.[81, 82]The combined fallout from all of these events contained certain types of radionuclides that will remain a threat to our food chain for well over 300 years (137Cs and 90Sr), and even for tens or hundreds of thousands of years (Technetium-99 (99Te) and Plutonium-239).[83] Indeed, from 1944 to 1962, the world was required to absorb 40,000 times more radiation than the amount released from the A-bomb dropped on Hiroshima.[84]

The original warnings came from physicists, such as Linus Pauling (1962 Nobel Peace Prize winner), Andrei D. Sakharov (1950s; later a 1975 Peace Nobel Prize winner) and Dr. Helen Caldicott, (founder of Physicians for Social Responsibility, an organization that won the Noble Peace Prize in 1985), who stated that in the decades ahead this nuclear fallout would kill millions and could easily cause germ mutations, creating massive deaths unlinked to their real cause, as well as unprecedented legions of super germs.[85, 86, 87, 88]

Fallout Spurs Contagion

Just as predicted, alarming emerging evidence suggests the Fukushima Catastrophe has indeed greatly fueled contagion throughout Japan. This should come as no surprise. Back in 1997 Dr. Alice Stewart reported that large numbers of WWII Japanese A-bomb survivors fell victim to a variety of infectious diseases.[89] Currently, the National Institute of Infectious Disease has documented dramatic increases in several infectious diseases for the time period starting after June of 2011. Each infectious disease rate that spiked on or after June of 2011 is charted, for comparison, onto the historical year-by-year infectious rates from 2001 to the present. For example, dramatic escalations have recently been seen for bacterial meningitis,[90] erythema infectiosum,[91] hand, foot and mouth disease,[92] mycoplasma pneumonia,[93] respiratory syncytial virus (RSV) infection,[94] and possibly for shigellosis/dysentery as well.[95]

With all of this emerging evidence, it makes anyone wonder if the sudden surge in outbreaks of food poisoning in regions known to have received radioactive fallout from the Fukushima Catastrophe, namely both in North America as well as in Europe, were not somehow related to this phenomenon unfolding in Japan.[96] Many of the outbreaks were tracked down to highly popular salad sprouts. Could the key have been unsuspected radionuclide contaminated water used to germinate the sprouts? In my neck of the woods in the U.S. NW, several sprout farms were shut down over this outbreak, and our entire region's water supply is well documented to have received significant fallout (see next chapter for complete details).

Uses of Radioactive Waste

Since the advent of nuclear energy, man has been looking for ways to productively use radioactive waste. Unfortunately, many decisions have been made without scientific evaluation and without full knowledge or disclosure about the impact of ingested radioactive materials on the human body. For instance, on November 16, 1987 thousands of acres of Oklahoma farmland were intentionally fertilized by aerial spraying of radioactive-laced fertilizer according to the *Wichita Falls Times Record News* in an article entitled, "Nuclear Waste Being Sprayed in Oklahoma." Here is the original report from *The New York Times*:

> *The Kerr-McGee Corporation, after years of tests and studies, is spraying thousands of acres of pastureland in eastern Oklahoma with a fertilizer recycled from radioactive wastes. The fertilizer, which the company describes as treated raffinate...contains nitrogen, trace amounts of radioactive uranium, radium and thorium, some toxic solvents and at least 18 potentially poisonous heavy metals, including arsenic, lead, mercury, molybdenum, nickel, cobalt and cadmium.*[97]
>
> *Kerr-McGee scientists say the levels of radioactive elements and most of the heavy metals in the fertilizer are equal to or lower than the amount in some commercial phosphate fertilizers...Still, many residents have called on the state and Federal governments to halt the spraying program, citing deaths of farm animals they cannot explain, several instances of gross malformations in newborn livestock and the discovery of a nine-legged frog in a pond that drains a pasture sprayed with treated raffinate. In high concentrations, radioactivity and some of the heavy metals are known to cause mutations, paralysis and even death...*

Fallout Arriving in Our Ports

Even more diabolical, the United States has unwittingly and now even wittingly imported vast quantities of radioactively contaminated foodstuffs and other materials into our marketplace.[98] Writing for Scripps Howard News Service, Isaac Wolf reported that:

> *Thousands of everyday products and materials containing radioactive metals are surfacing across the United States and around the world. Common kitchen cheese graters, reclining chairs, women's handbags and tableware manufactured with contaminated metals have been identified, some after having been in circulation for as long as a decade. So have fencing wire and fence posts, shovel blades, elevator buttons, airline parts and steel used in construction. A Scripps Howard News Service investigation has found that – because of haphazard screening, an absence of oversight and substantial disincentives for businesses to report contamination – no one knows how many tainted goods are in circulation in the United States. But thousands of consumer goods and millions of pounds of unfinished metal and its byproducts have been found to contain low levels of radiation, and experts think the true amount could be much higher, perhaps by a factor of 10.*[99]

Apparently, Secretary of State, Hillary Clinton, made a deal with the Japanese Prime Minister to protect world trade and Japan's economy after the Fukushima incident.[100] Japan's exports throughout the world would be declared perfectly safe and assumed not to be contaminated by radioactivity.[101, 102] Hopefully, the scope of this agreement will not deter ethical minded Food and Drug Administration (FDA) inspectors from continually scanning for radioactive contamination of Japanese goods arriving onto United States' soil as they have been since March 22nd, 2011.[103]

What concerns me most is that the FDA will use the less conservative derived intervention levels (or DIL) measurement scale to evaluate foodstuffs imported from Japan. This enables low doses of radioactive substances to enter into U.S. food supplies, which will trigger the "Petkau Effect" and the "bystander effect." These three all-important subjects (DIL, Petkau Effect, and bystander effect) are topics of great interest and will be discussed next. Furthermore, the FDA states they will restrict their most thorough testing to foodstuffs arriving from Japan to only three of its prefectures.[104] We now know food and water contamination has extended far beyond three prefectures.[105] For example, according to the Ministry of Education and Science, beef products in Japan have now contaminated the food supply with radioactive cesium in 296 schools in 12 prefectures.[106]

High-Dose Versus Low-Dose Radiation Exposure

Researchers from University of North Carolina School of Public Health and State University of New York School of Public Health published a rigorously peer-reviewed report about what actually happens in human populations after releases of radiation too low to "conceivably" cause any harm. They comment that there is a pervasive unfounded scientific bias that "believes" extremely low doses of radiation cannot correlate to the causality of escalations in cancer rates. Notwithstanding, the researchers meticulously document significant escalations in cancer rates in the surrounding areas of dozens of normally operating nuclear power plants from around the globe, and especially from here in the U.S. after the Three Mile Island crisis of 1979. [107, 108] This body of data has withstood the test of time, and clearly demonstrates causality despite repeated reports to the contrary. A very common flaw to these contrary reports was a clear "bending" or ignoring of the actual observed facts. The researchers described the inane and unsupportable contrarian bias this way:

> *"The only scientific reason to conduct studies of cancer around nuclear facilities is to evaluate whether radiation doses to neighboring populations result in a detectable increase in cancer risk. It is not logical to test a hypothesis of elevated cancer near facilities if it is decided a priori that results cannot be interpreted as evidence in support of the hypothesis. Such an exercise would amount to a public relations effort masquerading as a scientific study."*[109]

The Petkau Effect

Scientists differ on their statements regarding the impact of long term exposure to low dose radiation versus the impact of a one-time high dose exposure. Sakharov theorized that long-term low-dose radiation poisoning would do the greatest harm. Sakharov's theories were confirmed in 1971 by Dr. Abram Petkau,[110] working for the Canadian Atomic Energy Establishment in Pinowa, Manitoba. Petkau determined that the lethal implications of low-dose radiation were due to their effect on cellular lipid membranes (i.e., via creating widespread lipid peroxides or internal "fat-borne" ROS), in stark contrast to the belief that most of the lethal aspects to radiation poisoning affect genetic integrity.[111] His work was so monumental that this phenomenon is now called the "Petkau Effect." More recently, Petkau's discovery has been confirmed by experts familiar with his pioneering research.[112, 113]

The Bystander Effect

Fat-borne ROS (i.e., phosphorylated proteins) and other ROS melted or burned cell components also induce a "bystander effect." The bystander effect occurs when nearby cells, that are not directly exposed to ionizing radiation, are nevertheless destroyed.[114] The cells directly dosed with the radiation release ROS and/or highly proinflammatory cell end-products are capable of inducing a lethal chain reaction into surrounding nearby cells not directly exposed to the low-dose radiation.[115, 116] The amount of ROS and associated proinflammatory end-products can be so overwhelming, that non-exposed cells rapidly implode.[117] It now appears that these collective chemicals greatly influence the genetic core of the cells standing nearby as well.[118, 119] This suggests that the bystander effect may be a yet unrecognized extension of the Petkau Effect.

Both the Petkau Effect and bystander effect are brought on by low doses of radiation, and both can cause massive cell and tissue damage. One difference noted to date is that the low doses of radiation associated with the Petkau Effect are understood in the context of longer time periods than those currently associated with the bystander effect. Regardless, the bystander effect, even if it arises over short time frames, is likely contributory to the more comprehensive Petkau Effect. Surprisingly, "very low" doses of radiation are more toxic than doses that most consider to be "low."[120]

Interestingly, cell-to-cell signals sent between the exposed and non-exposed cells appear to also enable regeneration of the hardiest cells under circumstances not yet clearly defined.[121] However, because of the generation of particles called "micronuclei" consistent with autophagy (a form of cell repair system that can also self-select for cell death if stresses are too great), this likely explains at least in part the observed cellular regeneration.[122, 123] This is important to note because later in this book, great importance is given to how the process of autophagy will help regenerate your tissues after exposure to radiation, especially when properly supported by select nutrients.

What is the potential impact of low-dose radiation which spurs both the Petkau Effect as well as the bystander effect? Since 1970, the worldwide low-dose exposure to radioactive fallout has again climbed via the release of more than 370 trillion picocuries of radioactive iodine, strontium, cesium and other elements. The consequences were a dramatic rise in the United States death rate associated with cancer and immune deficiency.[124] In large measure, these constant low-level releases are due to the regular releases from nuclear power plants. Unfortunately, these releases as mentioned above are an established practice of nuclear power plant operations.[125]

The Transgenerational Threat to Humankind and All Life on Earth

For decades, many nuclear scientists, industry engineers and health physicists mistakenly believed that in general the shorter the given half-life of a high energy emitting radionuclide, the more dangerous it is. [126] For example, radioactive depleted uranium (DU) is used in military arsenals. DU is an ideal armor-piercing heavy metal when fashioned into a shell or missile warhead. During impact, it vaporizes into a finely powdered dust that scatters into the local biosphere. DU has a half-life of 4.5 billion years, so it is an extremely slow emitter of ionizing radiation. Yet, the dust from DU weapons explosions becomes immediately devastating and commonly lethal to all exposed life forms.[127]

For those with a proclivity toward science, the power of the Petkau Effect may be best described with the following.[128, 129]

A long-term exposure of extremely low radiation (i.e., one-ten millionth of a rad per minute) was found to be 100 BILLION times MORE lethal than a short-term exposure to exceedingly high level radiation (i.e., 10,000 rads per minute). As it turns out, Petkau discovered that at exceedingly high radiation levels, the abundant ROS generated in tissues tended to cancel each other out before they could do cellular damage. But at extremely low radiation levels, these same free radicals - produced in minuscule quantities - remain unchecked. And any steady stream of unchecked ROS will efficiently and lethally cleave lipid cellular membranes like a hot knife slicing through butter once they overwhelm and exhaust cellular antioxidant defenses. This dramatically illustrates the non-linear aspects of dose (rads) to lethality. Many scientists specializing in the field of nuclear medicine are unaware of the new data substantiating this fact, unless they are keeping up with more recent studies on "bystander effects."

Indeed, the impact of radiation poisoning delineated by the Petkau Effect is the most alarming to me as a physician due to its capacity to cause human debilitation and even death thousands of miles away. The Petkau Effect overrides all of my other concerns because the radioactive fallout in North America caused by the Fukushima Daiichi Nuclear Power Plant disaster leads to incessant, long term low-dose radiation poisoning from a fleet of radionuclides sporting half-lives from days to billions of years! Americans simply can't run, and they can't hide from this catastrophe. So, understanding this concept is essential to thinking about how to protect ourselves now and for many decades ahead. Our biggest challenge is to understand that protection from radiation fallout must be accomplished in such a way that it neutralizes both the Petkau Effect as well as the longer-term effects of radiation upon genetic mutations. In Chapter 4, I explain how these two strategies must be integrated.

As a matter of fact, modern society – that society produced by science and technology – is committing the same mistake as have all the civilizations of antiquity. It has created conditions of life wherein life itself becomes impossible. It justifies the sally of Dean Inge: "Civilization is a disease which is almost invariably fatal."

Alexis Carrel in *Man the Unknown*

Chapter Two

Fukushima Daiichi Nuclear Power Plant

To help you more precisely understand the global health impact of the radionuclide release at Fukushima, let me detail the explosive events that occurred due to the earthquake and resulting tsunami. Even more interesting is the overview I provide of the radionuclides and how they travel through the atmosphere. Finally, I'll discuss the current radioactive measurements systems including the amount in water and milk in Japan and the United States. We'll start by focusing on:

- The design and composition of the nuclear fuel rod itself.
- The dispersal and penetration of the radioactivity locally, globally and into human tissues.[130]
- Types of radioactive elements released at Fukushima

The Fuel Rod

Imagine a hollow metal pole twelve feet long. Next, imagine radioactive uranium pellets all the size of peanuts with shells intact. These pellets are packed into that hollow metal tube. This hollow metal pole and the uranium inside are called a fuel rod that is made in part of a material called Zircaloy, from zirconium. There are thousands of these 12-foot long fuel rods inside a nuclear reactor.

Under normal circumstances, nuclear fission inside these fuel rods causes heat that boils water which makes steam that in turn makes electricity. But, the nuclear fission also creates radioactive daughter products (i.e., daughter radionuclides) that also generate heat. And the build-up of these daughter radionuclides escalates to the point that they must be released by design or by accident, and therein lays the problem. Even when the nuclear power plant is operating normally, it must release these pent-up daughter radionuclides. But in an accident, vastly higher amounts are released into the surrounding regions. There are hundreds of these daughter radionuclides, including 131-I, 90Sr and 137Cs. A combination of coolant swirling around these rods and other control measures keeps the uranium from melting through its containment.

There are typically two layers of containment shielding the fuel rods from the outer environment. The collective fuel rods (or nuclear reactor core) are enclosed in their own containment called a reactor vessel. This shielding is tough but thinner than the secondary, thicker outer containment structure. Due to the incoming and outgoing attachments to this reactor vessel, another outer 3 meter thick containment structure is constructed in such a way to, in theory, seal in the nuclear reactor core if meltdown conditions are underway during an accident.

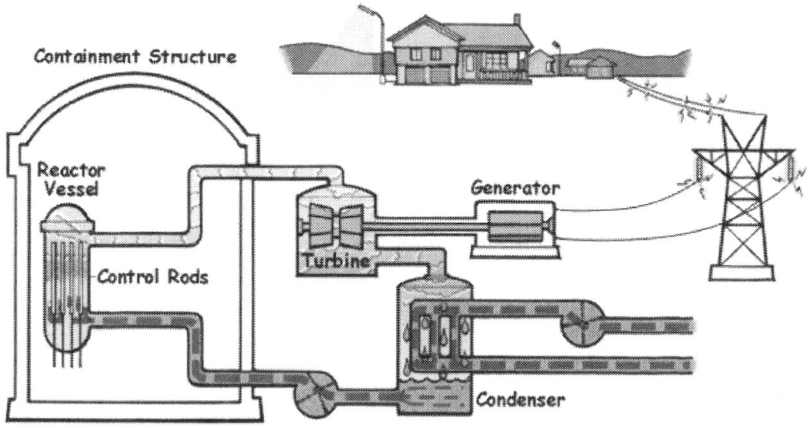

Figure 2.1: Boiling Water Reactor (BWR) of a Nuclear Power Plant
Source: U.S. Nuclear Regulatory Commission (NRC)[131]

During an accident, four possible critical events stand out:

1. Partial Meltdown

2. Complete Meltdown

3. Reactor Vessel Melt-Through

4. A China Syndrome

Partial Meltdown

When coolant stops swirling around the fuel rods and other control measures fail in an accident, extreme heat production and even uncontrolled chain reactions (fission) may continue for a long time. Under these circumstances, the cooling water will begin to rapidly boil turning into super-heated, highly pressurized steam. At this point, the water loses most of its ability to cool the fuel rods from overheating. As the fuel rods continue to overheat, each fuel rod approaches meltdown temperatures. If this continues, incremental "Meltdown" of the fuel rods may begin. The scenario goes something like this. The heat of the fuel rods gradually escalates upward, first above 300°C, then 500°C and then even up toward 1,200°C. As the fuel rods heat up, their Zircaloy content may begin to react with the steam to create explosive hydrogen gas, which is a chemical reaction. Now this becomes a full-blown crisis.

The higher the temperature rises, the more dangerous things become. For example, as the temperature rises toward the upper extreme:

1. The risk of a hydrogen explosion becomes greater and greater.
2. The amount of super heated steam becomes greater and greater.
3. Pooling of the molten blob grows and grows into pools at the bottom of the reactor vessel
4. Vapors of highly lethal daughter products, such as 137Cs, climb.

Complete Meltdown

The following leads to a complete meltdown. In addition to the formation of super-heated, highly pressurized steam and hydrogen gas, two other dangers arise during the meltdown. As more and more of the fuel rods melt, the internal uranium pellets may begin to pool together into a 'molten blob' at the base of the fuel rod racks, which up until now held all fuel rods within the reactor vessel.

The uranium pellets within the fuel rods begin to melt, releasing more and more radioactive daughter products. At 1,000°C, 137Cs is 100% volatilized (fully vaporized) after one hour;[132] and at 2,467°C (2740°K), 137Cs is 100% volatilized after 40 minutes.[133] As the temperatures hit 1,500°C, then 2,000°C and finally up to 2,760°C (5,000°F), complete melt-down temperatures have been attained.

Reactor Vessel Melt-Through

With enough pressurized steam, pressurized hydrogen gas and pooling of super-heated blobs at the bottom of the reactor vessel, the reactor vessel containment may rupture. If the rupture occurs at the bottom of the reactor vessel where the super-heated blob has collected, this is called a melt-through. Eventually the super-heated water coolant evaporates or leaks out of the crippled reactor vessel's containment and the fuel rods become exposed to open air. Along with the steam, vapors of the daughter products travel out to the open air.

Once vaporized, the 137Cs is in the ideal state to more completely contaminate the outside biosphere, especially if it is liberated via an explosion of some kind. Reactor Units 1-3 at the Fukushima Daiichi Nuclear Power Plant all experienced both partial to complete meltdown of their respective reactor nuclear cores as well as reactor vessel melt-throughs.

The China Syndrome

If the molten blob which has fallen to the inside bottom of the outer containment structure were to melt through this last containment layer, by definition this would be The China Syndrome. There is no evidence to date to indicate The China Syndrome has occurred at the Fukushima Daiichi Nuclear Power Plant. This fact remains as of October 7th, 2011, even though there have been unprecedented releases of solid, liquid and vaporized radioactive materials into the local, regional and global biosphere.

Explosive Potential of Melting Fuel Rods

Fuel rods can be damaged through melting or through explosions. When Zircaloy fuel rods are subjected to extreme temperatures, it becomes possible for the fuel rods to spontaneously ignite, creating even more heat. Such temperatures occur if the fuel rods become exposed to air for enough time. This condition drives partial or complete meltdown of the fuel core.[134]

Zircaloy plus steam naturally creates more heat at all temperatures. At 1,200°C, large amounts of hydrogen may form according to the following equation:

Steam + Zircaloy ➔ Zircaloy oxide + Hydrogen

Written as: $2(H_2O) + Zr \rightarrow ZrO_2 + 2(H_2)$

The resulting production of vast amounts of hydrogen is itself a potential source for an explosion. Just one spark and Ka-Blamm!

Once the temperature proceeds unabated to approximately 1500°C (2732°F), the rate of heat/hydrogen generation dramatically skyrockets. Providing there is a reserve of oxygen and the heat is not transferred away from the Zircaloy, the reaction will not terminate until all Zircaloy is consumed. In other words, at 1500°C and above, the chemical reactions are self-sustaining until all the Zircaloy is consumed and the bundles of reactor fuel rods no longer exist because they melt down into a molten blob.

In the final stages of a full meltdown of nuclear reactor core, temperatures may approach 2,760°C (5,000°F). During this uncontrolled self-sustaining temperature escalation, the daughter radionuclides like 131-I, 90Sr and 137Cs in the fuel rods rapidly vaporize.[135, 136] Any vaporized (volatilized) radionuclides become extremely dangerous since, if an explosion occurs, they go airborne and may travel great distances. Three kinds of explosions can instantly cause either the reactor vessel to breach, or the outer structure containment to breach, or both. These are:

- A sub-sonic explosion or "deflagration"
- A super-sonic explosion or "detonation"
- A nuclear detonation

Each kind of explosion escalates the potential danger to humanity, with a nuclear detonation being the most severe. The underlying energy to these three kinds of explosions is improperly controlled or uncontrolled nuclear chain reactions. An improperly controlled chain reaction may produce the conditions for: (a) an explosive chemical reaction, (b) a vapor explosion, (c) a combination of the two, or (d) a pure conversion of radioactive materials into explosive amounts of pure energy.

Deflagration

A sub-sonic explosion is called a deflagration. A sub-sonic chemical explosion would occur at lower temperatures (~500°C up to 1,500°C) that could generate sufficient hydrogen gas via the following equation: $2(H_2O) + Zr \rightarrow ZrO_2 + 2(H_2)$. At some point, this hydrogen gas (which is highly flammable) comes into contact with a spark, and there is an explosion.[137] A deflagration would tend to send less radioactivity beyond the boundaries of the nuclear power plant.

A deflagration happened at Fukushima Unit 1 building, which blew the roof clean-off, thereby spewing radiation into the local biosphere. The source of the explosive hydrogen gas appears to have come from the Unit 1 reactor vessel, which leaked the gas up into the ceiling of the Unit 1 building. The Unit 1 storage fuel pool was likely not involved in this deflagration. The Unit 4 storage fuel pool likely had its own deflagration.

Reactor vessels have valves to enable gases to escape to prevent rupturing the primary containment around the reactor vessel. Later it appears that the primary containment did breach in a separate incident, perhaps involving a melt-through, a chemical reaction, a vapor explosion, or some combination. Additionally, the Unit 2 reactor vessel suffered a breach from a valve adjoining the dry well with the wet well (torus).

In both cases, we simply may never know the exact sequence or combination of factors that caused all the destruction in Reactor Building Units 1, 2 and 4.[138] A deflagration which spews radionuclides creates a regional and national crisis.

Detonation

A supersonic explosion is called a "detonation." To produce a supersonic explosion, meltdown temperatures reach higher levels (+1,500°C) and thus it is associated with a more intense chain reaction called a moderated "prompt-criticality." Such a chain reaction would multiply itself a thousand times per second.

In any nuclear accident where moderated prompt-criticalities occur, one or more fuel rod assemblies may become super-heated due to coolant and/or control rod failure, and form a molten blob at the bottom of the fuel rod stacks. When this super-heated molten blob comes into contact with any remaining coolant, a supersonic explosion may ensue because the coolant-in-contact (or other moderating material) becomes unable to dissipate the extreme heat fast enough in any other fashion.[139]

A moderated prompt-criticality detonation changes the catastrophe from a national or regional emergency into a global emergency.[140] The supersonic explosion that occurred in Chernobyl Reactor 4 is one example of what happens in a well-fueled moderated prompt criticality. The explosion at the Fukushima Unit 3 (storage fuel pool and/or reactor vessel) is another example of a supersonic detonation that was even more powerful than Chernobyl's.

Such detonations would send a broad-spectrum array of radioactive elements in vastly more lethal amounts (including plutonium) high into the atmosphere and around the globe than a less energetic deflagration explosion. In a separate incident, the reactor vessel's primary containment at Unit 3 became breached, likely from a melt-through or a combination of a vapor and/or chemical explosion, allowing radioactive steam to spew about the biosphere. We may simply never know its exact cause.[141]

Nuclear Detonation

A nuclear detonation arises when the chain reaction escalates to where it is multiplying itself a million times per second, or approximately three orders of magnitude more than a moderated prompt-criticality detonation.[142, 143] As of August 2011, a nuclear detonation is not thought to have occurred at Fukushima.

Fukushima experienced both deflagrations and detonations, which means that Japan is now in real trouble. During the Chernobyl explosion, the radioactive plume was vaulted 2.5 kilometers into the air,[144] but during the Fukushima explosions, the radioactive plume was vaulted 5 kilometers into the air due to a low pressure system passing over eastern Japan at that time.[145]

Once the denial mentality begins to wane at the official levels of the Japanese government, it should become apparent that vast territories within the nation of Japan may be uninhabitable. Already all the signs of widespread contamination are appearing. For example, on May 1st, the Fukushima Prefectural Government announced that alarmingly high levels of 137Cs were detected in sewage sludge at a purification center in Koriyama, Fukushima Prefecture. More alarming detections of 137Cs in sludge showed up at 15 other sewage plants in the prefecture, as well as at sewage treatment facilities in Tochigi Prefecture, Ibaraki Prefecture, Gunma Prefecture and Niigata Prefecture. Then, less than two weeks later, the Kanagawa Prefectural Government announced that cesium was detected in four more sewage plants, while the Tokyo Metropolitan Government disclosed the same day that high levels of radioactivity were detected at three more sewage plants in the capital.[146] Measurable 137Cs has been found in the urine of children and adults in the region. Fish and whales have also been tested positive for 137Cs.

Radioactive Fallout from Fukushima

How much radiation was really released from Fukushima? No one will ever know, because all of the instruments to measure radiation were either destroyed by the explosions or lost electricity to operate. Therefore, our best estimates can only be derived from advanced simulation technology.[147] Like Chernobyl before it, scientists and engineers try to calculate how much they think was released. A key to these calculations is the assumptions the engineers choose to use. The Japanese owners of Fukushima Daiichi Nuclear Power Plant (TEPCO,

Tokyo Electric Power Company) have already modified their prediction multiple times, each time stating that the amount of radiation was worse than the previous estimate. It is in the best interest of the Japanese officials to minimize these release estimates by choosing assumptions that lower the releases.

Independent scientists at Woods Hole Oceanographic Institute have stated that radioactive releases from Fukushima into the Pacific Ocean are ten times higher than Chernobyl.[148] Other independent scientists have questioned a key assumption; exactly how much 137Cs was trapped in the water inside the containment? The Japanese have assumed that 99% of the 137Cs remains trapped in the water, but scientists outside of Japan have noted that this water was boiling and could not have captured much 137Cs. In fact, data suggests that boiling water captures *no* 137Cs. These independent scientists believe that 137Cs releases were in fact much worse than Chernobyl.

So how much radiation really was released? Scientifically, we must rely on ocean and land measurements, plus computer simulations. Unscientifically stated, it is bad, really bad.

The International Atomic Energy Agency (IAEA) has identified dangerously high radiation levels 25 miles to the west and northwest of the Fukushima Daiichi Nuclear Power Plant. These levels exceed (by a factor of four) the levels of radioactivity that set the boundaries of the "exclusion zone" around Chernobyl.[149] Chernobyl's exclusion zone extends outward 19 miles in all directions from the single nuclear reactor that blew. Chernobyl's "exclusion zone" is the zone that has been declared uninhabitable, and will remain so for tens if not hundreds of years.

The implication of the regional Fukushima contamination levels being four times higher than that of Chernobyl's exclusion zone implies that it may be too risky for families to live within 100 miles to the west and northwest of the Fukushima Daiichi Nuclear Power Plant for tens if not hundreds of years.[150]

I developed Table 2.1 to construct a working draft for the purpose of gauging and appraising the levels of fallout we might expect from the Fukushima Catastrophe. I created a set of reasonable assumptions based in part from the historical experience of the Chernobyl Catastrophe. It took the International Atomic Energy Agency (IAEA) and the Organization for Economic Co-Operation and Development (OECD) 10 years to produce final data computations on Chernobyl that have withstood the test of time. So, we can expect these projections to undergo a revision process for at least as long. In the meantime, we need them now to assess and consider all reasonable means to protect ourselves and our children from this day forward.

Table 2.1 Comparative Estimate of Fukushima Regional and Global Fallout: Next 20 Years or More[151, 152, 153, 154, 155]

Radio-nuclide	Half-life	Biological Impact	Chernobyl Catastrophe	Fukushima Catastrophe	Atmospheric Bomb Tests	Hanford
33Xe	5.3 days	53 days	$6,500X10^{15}Bq$	$45,500X10^{15}Bq$		$15X10^{15}Bq$
131-I	8 days	80 days	$3,200X10^{15}Bq$	$22,400X10^{15}Bq$	$650,000X10^{15}Bq$	$29X10^{15}Bq$
134Cs	2 years	20 years	$180X10^{15}Bq$	$1,260X10^{15}Bq$		
137Cs	30 years	300 years	$280X10^{15}Bq$	$1,960X10^{15}Bq$	$912X10^{15}Bq$	
89Sr	52 days	520 days	$2,300X10^{15}Bq$	$16,100X10^{15}Bq$		
90Sr	28 years	280 years	$200X10^{15}Bq$	$1,400X10^{15}Bq$	$604X10^{15}Bq$	$17X10^{15}Bq$
106Ru	1 year	10 years	$2,100X10^{15}Bq$	$14,700X10^{15}Bq$		
238Pu	86 years	860 years	$1X10^{15}Bq$	$7 X10^{15}Bq$		
239Pu	24,400 yrs	244,000 yrs	$0.85X10^{15}Bq$	$5.95X10^{15}Bq$	$6.5 X10^{15}Bq$	$233X10^{15}Bq$
240Pu	6,580 yrs	65,800 yrs	$1.2X10^{15}Bq$	$8.4 X10^{15}Bq$	$4.4 X10^{15}Bq$	
241Pu	13.2 yrs	132 yrs	$170 X10^{15}Bq$	$1,190 X10^{15}Bq$	$142 X10^{15}Bq$	
Totals			$12,000X10^{15}Bq$	$84,000X10^{15}Bq$	$+1,000,000X10^{15}Bq$	$16,169X10^{15}Bq$

ASSUMPTIONS:

- Total weight per fuel rod assembly = 320kg per fuel rod, or 700lbs (or 0.35 tons) per fuel rod.[156]
- Chernobyl: Grand total Unit 4 reactor initial load which was exposed to meltdown conditions = 190 tons, of which 70% or 135 tons was destroyed (i.e., melted, volatilized or burned), and was released into the global biosphere.[157]
- Fukushima: Grand total nuclear materials released into greater environment = 954 tons.
- 954/135 = seven times Chernobyl 12,000 X 10^{15} Bq[158] ➔ 84,000 X 10^{15} Bq released into the greater environment, through (a) volatilization, (b) steam releases, (c) ground water/water table, and (d) oceanic releases over the next 20 years.
- Timeline for 100% release and impact into the general biosphere for all fission daughter products: (a) first 50% impacting the next 20 years, and the remaining 50% impacting (b) the following 80 years thereafter (due to decay of respective radionuclide half-life and bioaccumulation/biomagnification into regional and global food chains).
- These estimations do not account for the increased inventories of 137Cs and 90Sr, expected in the older spent fuel rods. Inclusion of such inventories could "spike" 137Cs and 90Sr levels noted below by a considerable margin.[159]
- Fukushima: Unit 4 building remains intact and its storage fuel pool (SFP) radioactive contents have not been destroyed in excess of 40% at the time of this writing (July 10th, 2011).

- Fukushima: Units 1 and 2 SFP radioactive contents experienced approximately 5% damage to their fuel rod contents.

- Miscellaneous data points for Fukushima Daiichi Nuclear Power Plant:
  - Unit 4 SFP = 1,535 assemblies[160, 161] X 0.35 = ~537 tons of fuel ~40% burned...[162, 163] = ~215 tons.
  - Unit 3 SFP = 566 assemblies[164] X 0.35 = ~198 tons of fuel ~100% destroyed = ~198 tons.
  - Unit 3 Reactor Core = 548 assemblies[165] X 0.35 = ~192 tons of fuel ~100% melted...[166] = ~192 tons.
  - Unit 2 SFP = 615 assemblies[167] X 0.35 = ~215 tons of fuel ~5% released...[168] = ~10 tons.
  - Unit 2 Reactor Core = 548 assemblies[169] X 0.35 = ~192 tons of fuel @ 100% melted...[170] = ~192 tons.
  - Unit 1 SFP = 392 assemblies[171] X 0.35 = ~137 tons of fuel ~5% released...~ 7 tons.
  - Unit 1 Reactor Core = 400 assemblies[172] X 0.35 = ~140 tons of fuel ~100% melted...[173] = ~140 tons.
- Grand Total Damaged Nuclear Fuel @ Fukushima Daiichi Catastrophe = ~954 tons.
- Grand Total Damaged Nuclear Fuel @ Chernobyl Catastrophe = ~135 tons.
- Fukushima :: Chernobyl Radioactive Release Ratio = ~7::1
- Fukushima :: Chernobyl *Regional* Population Ratio exposed to >4 kBq/m2[174,175, 176, 177, 178, 179, 180, 181, 182] = ~6::1
- Fukushima Catastrophe *Regional* Impact Ratio (7 times more Radiation x 6 times more population) = 42 times Chernobyl Catastrophe

Confirmation has Already Begun

The projection or forecast of the "Fukushima to Chernobyl Radioactive Release Ratio" (i.e., 7::1) will be fully realized over the coming decades as groups of internationally recognized experts track the outcome. Even today, such signs are apparent.

The International Nuclear and Radiological Event Scale (INES) was used to make final calculations comparing the Fukushima Catastrophe to Chernobyl during *the first eleven days* of the crisis (the time period from March 12th, 2011 through March 22nd, 2011). The data consisted of fallout of both 131-I as well as 137Cs. Two authoritative and independent agencies collected this data: the French Institut de Radioprotection et de Sûreté Nucléaire (IRSN) (www.irsn.fr), which published an estimation covering reactor Units 1 through 3; and the Austrian Zentralanstalt für Meteorologie und Geodynamik (ZAMG) (www.zamg.ac.at), which published estimations covering the total release of 131-I and 137Cs during *the first four days* of the crises.

According to the INES, the Chernobyl Catastrophe released an amount of radiation rated as a 7, on a scale of 1 to 7, where 1 is the lowest, and 7 is the highest. This data pertaining to *the first eleven days* release of radioactive fallout from the Fukushima Daiichi Nuclear Power Plant was then conservatively rated on the INES scale. The data clearly indicates that just from *the initial eleven days* after the earthquake, the Fukushima Catastrophe released a plume of radioactivity equivalent to *three* – INES Scale 7 events![183]

The above calculations are based upon levels of both 131-I and 137Cs. But we also have a reliable data base on another radioactive fallout emission common to nuclear power plant accidents, namely for xenon-133 (133Xe). A recent article calculated that the Pacific NW experienced exposures to 133Xe that were 40,000 higher than the average to this area.[184]

Using this data point, it becomes possible to compare the total release of 133Xe experienced during the Chernobyl Catastrophe to the total Fukushima release up to March 16th. The comparison suggests that as of March 16th, 2011, the world received from two to five times more radioactive fallout from the Fukushima Catastrophe than it did during the entire Chernobyl Catastrophe.[185]

We are not holding our breath awaiting comprehensive reports from government or United Nation agencies who are tracing, but under reporting, the total air, sea, land and water table releases from Fukushima since March 22nd.[186, 187]

It should be noted that despite all the evidence showing that the Fukushima Catastrophe will far outpace that of the Chernobyl Catastrophe, the Nuclear Regulatory Agency (NRC) has decided to downgrade how it estimates death rates from reactor accidents. Scientists and nuclear watchdog groups are already commenting that the recent NRC report may be guilty of "bending science."[188]

Bending Science in Radioactive Reporting

The Fukushima Catastrophe may have resulted in a situation where officials became obsessed with bending science. In the Introduction to their book, *Bending Science*, Professors of Law Thomas O. McGarity and Wendy E. Wagner provide us with information regarding reliability of the modern scientific process:

For quite a while now, judges, legal scholars, and prominent scientists have lamented the difficulties that courts and lawmakers encounter in distinguishing reliable science from cleverly manipulated, but ultimately worthless scientific junk. Inundated by experts-for-hire who flood the legal system selling their sponsor's wares, legal decision-makers have struggled to develop more rigorous tools for assessing the reliability of the scientific information that informs health policies...Yet the simple solution of deferring to the scientists can be frustrating for legal decision-makers and even more precarious for the institutions of science. Accounts of 'bending' science – where research is manipulated to advance economic or ideological ends – are now not only prevalent in the corridors of courts and legislatures, but also beginning to emerge from deep within the inner sanctum of science.[189]

Suspect Data from the Environmental Protection Agency

On a blog frequented by students at UC Berkeley's Department of Physics, questions were raised on the Fukushima Catastrophe related to United States Environmental Protection Agency (EPA) data presented in Chart 2.1 below. Why are the pre-earthquake tracings so much higher than the post-earthquake tracings? Why the unexplainable decrease in the amplitude of the tracings on March 11th? One would expect that as radiation began arriving onto United States' soils by March 18th, spikes much higher than the pre-earthquake recordings would become readily apparent. Yet, upon close examination, it is almost as if someone decided to recalibrate the Sacramento tracings down by one or more orders of magnitude of their original calibration. The blogger on Berkeley's Nuclear Engineering website noted that upon reviewing tracings pertaining to other United States' regions monitored by the EPA, this same suspicious reduction in tracing amplitude likewise occurred.[190]

What caught my attention was that another nuclear engineering blogger on the same Berkeley website page, dated Sunday April 24th, 19:00, went on to speculate how peculiar it appeared to be that a name matching a former undersecretary of the Department of Interior was in charge of the nationwide radiation monitoring service for the EPA.[191] The blogger referred to a Patricia Bradshaw, President of Environmental Dimensions, Inc. (EDi). The same blogger alleged EDi may have been awarded the EPA radiation monitoring contract without any competitive bidding. This appeared to me to be a red flag. So, I started to dig into both EDi as well as the name Patricia Bradshaw.[192]

What I learned was indeed a bit chilling in implication. An EDi pdf states the following: "EDi is pleased to present the industry's first Automated Response Calibration Station (ARCS) technology. ARCS is specifically designed to automate the calibration process for radiation detection instrumentation."[193] Go figure. We can now clearly see that at the time of the Fukushima Catastrophe, by the simple push of a button, recalibrating the EPA's monitoring system was indeed technologically feasible.

Fortunately, having endured so much intrigue over fallout levels hitting NW America, we may now finally know the truth, the whole truth, and nothing but the truth. A recent study concluded that the actual fallout reaching NW America *was four to five orders of magnitude greater than* the levels occurring before the March 11th earthquake![194] Please note that the EPA data applicable to both Sacramento, California (shown below), as well as Seattle, WA, *do not reflect* such dramatic escalations in fallout.[195] This begs several questions - just who is responsible at the EPA for providing the American public with such shoddy data? Who is really running the EPA? And is it finally time to completely dismantle the EPA and start over again from scratch, only with built in mechanisms for preventing cronyism the next time around?

Suspect Data from the Japanese Ministry of Internal Affairs

Japan may have followed suit in this suspicious altering of radiation readings. A report appearing in Japan's premier business journal, authored by an expert in nuclear medicine, confirms that:

> *The release of data from the expensive SPEEDI system was delayed until March 23. This delay resulted in unnecessary radiation exposure. "It is only conceivable that the high rate of radiation released was not reported because of fears of a panic." The report goes on to say, "Former Minister for Internal Affairs Haraguchi Kazuhiro has alleged that radiation monitoring station data was actually three decimal places greater than the numbers released to the public. If this is true, it constitutes a 'national crime.... "*[196]

Perhaps future investigations (both in the U.S. as well as in Japan) into these unexplained reductions in tracing amplitudes will bring the matter to a credible conclusion.

Suspect Data from the Nuclear Regulatory Committee

Recent emails procured under the Freedom Of Information Act (FOIA) suggest certain members of the Nuclear Regulatory Commission do not want to be fully forthcoming to the American public. For example, one FOIA released email, sent on Tuesday, March 22nd 2011 at 7:49AM, with the subject heading: Tues 0730 - Commissioners Assistants Briefing on Japanese Events, reported that, "The Bounding Plausible Analysis, which needs peer review, would indicate elevated child thyroid dose to those in Midway Island and Alaska. This assumes 1 core and 2 SFPs released. (25% U2 Core, 50% U3 SFP, 100% U4 SFP)." This initial Bounding Plausible Analysis estimated up to 362 tons of radioactive fuel was damaged and was spreading its daughter products across the Pacific Ocean onto North American soils.

This data indicated three things:

- The children in Midway Island and Alaska were likely to become contaminated with enough cancer causing 131-I to be a concern.
- The officials knew of no antidotes to the absorbed 131-I and left the public in the dark.
- They failed to realize that more areas of North America were likely at risk and people could have at least been warned to take all prudent precautionary measures.

So instead of taking the initial Bounding Plausible Analysis seriously, why not simply have a policy in place that says to always err on the side of public safety? The response from the NRC officials was to shut down further communication. One official wrote, "No, they are not to be forwarded. They are full of speculation from many sources and are not to be quoted."[197] Well, what's the point of throwing together a "Bounding Plausible Analysis" anyway folks? For those interested, the Bounding Plausible Analysis is compiled by the best experts in the world (at NRC, NARAC, DOE, TEPCO, etc...) and involves mathematical equations that quantify the flow rate of accidental radiation releases into the environment (called the source term).

On Thursday of that same week an email originating from an NRC technical assistant updates the source(s) term as follows: "NRC, NARAC, DOE, others have agreed to a sources term for modeling the plausible bounding scenario with now no issue of SFP pool fire but more of a "super core" approach using 33% for Unit 1, 2, and 3 cores with fixed leak rate assumption. Effort done thru interagency working group..."[198] Although this update two days later cut in half the estimate of the sources term (from ~362 tons down to ~173 tons), the best experts in the world knew substantial releases of radioactivity had indeed occurred. Well, as it turns out both "Bounding Plausible Analyses" were low ball figures, by up to a factor of ~3. The best estimates to date I could find tally the "sources term" closer to 954 tons, confirming that North American kids clearly fell into harm's way.

Yet, as of October 8th, 2011, no final public draft of NRC's Bounding Plausible Analysis, with all the nitty, gritty details, has been forthcoming. So for the time being, let's move on to discuss the fallout time periods plotted against currently available data.

North American Radioactive Migration

Due to the Fukushima Catastrophe, North America has been inundated with radioactivity (fallout). Chart 2.1 was compiled by the Environmental Protection Agency (EPA).[199] It offers an interesting glimpse into our fate and raises suspicions regarding the integrity of the entire U.S. monitoring process. The question for the scientists to explain is: How did the radiation levels in Sacramento suddenly *drop* after the earthquake, while the Fukushima plant was spewing radioactivity into the atmosphere?

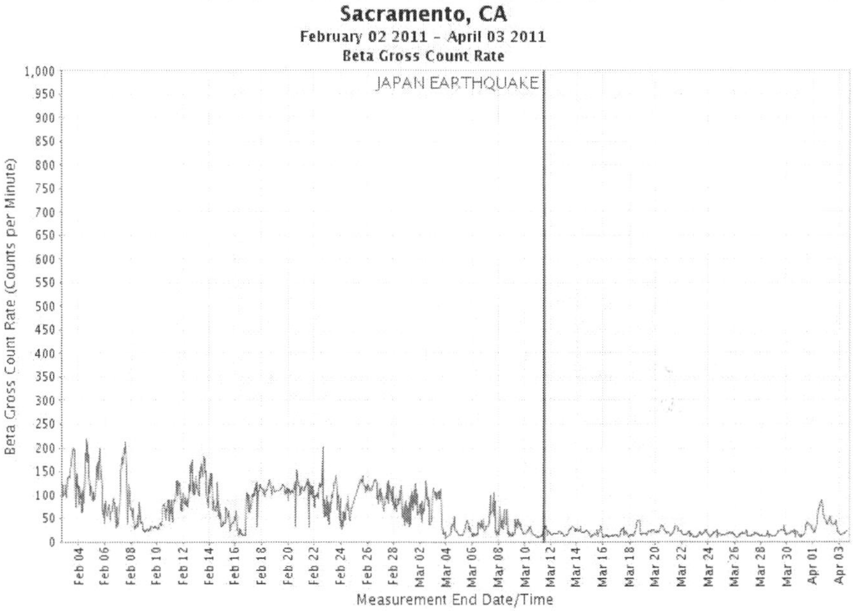

Chart 2.1 Radiation in Sacramento February 2 through April Source: Environmental Protection Agency (EPA)

Chart 2.2 shows additional EPA radiation recordings. Note the mysterious, non-continuous tracings, but only at exactly those points in time that record dramatic spikes in radiation. Notice that you can only see continuous tracings when the ratings are low. The EPA explains that the non-continuous line tracings were simply due to technical problems typical of their technology.[200]

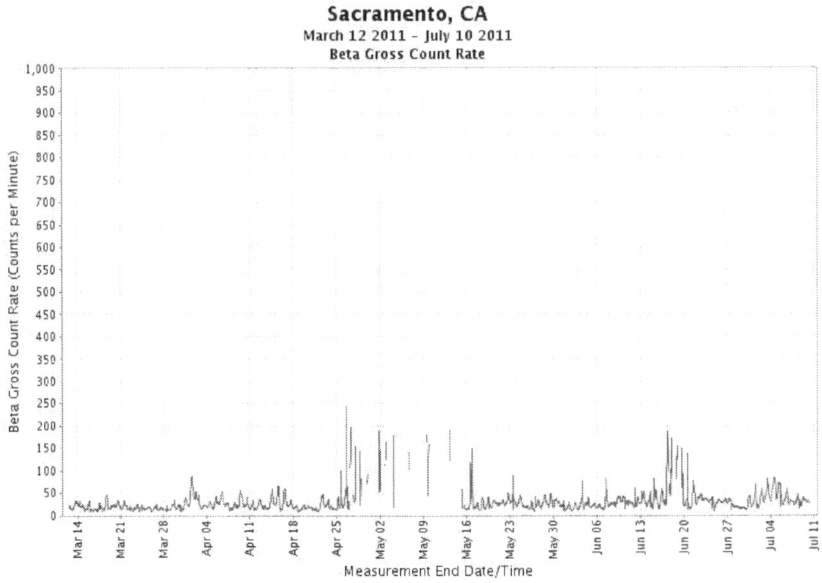

Chart 2.2 Radiation in Sacramento Mar 14 through Jul 11, 2011
Source: Environmental Protection Agency (EPA)

Timetables

Because the EPA charts do not give a clear picture, let's look at the data we do have to paint a clear picture. Rainstorms are the best catalyst for bringing radioactive particles to North American soils. Without rain, incoming airflows laced with radioactivity would arbitrarily skip over entire regions of the U.S.

There were massive releases of radiation into the upper atmosphere via several explosions at Fukushima Daiichi Nuclear Power Plant at the following times:

1. The first explosion (deflagration) occurred on March 12th at 3:36 PM at Fukushima's Unit 1 building.

2. A second massive explosion (detonation) at Unit 3 (reactor vessel or SFP?) occurred on March 14th at 11:00 AM. These releases of radioactivity were nothing compared to what was coming.

3. Unit 2 exploded on March 15th at 6:10 AM, almost at the exact time that Unit 4 exploded in fire. The fire at Unit 4 lasted for five hours, releasing vast amounts of radiation through the smoke. During the same time period as the fire raged at Unit 4, a second explosion occurred at Unit 2 at 10:00 AM.

4. At approximately 12:00 AM in the morning of March 16th, another massive and mysterious radiation release occurred.

5. Then, later that same day, Units 2 and 3 released the second largest amount of radiation recorded.

6. Late in the day of March 16th, the radiation started to taper off slowly until just before midnight of March 21st.

7. Sometime between 1:00 AM and 3:00 AM on March 21st, the pressure sky-rocketed to 110 atmospheres (~1,617 pounds per square inch![201]) within the Unit 3 reactor likely due to another explosion. If true, this may have led to round two of the core's meltdown, with subsequent release of more radiation to the general biosphere.

8. A spike of radiation once again rose on the morning of March 24th.[202, 203]

By the end of the third day after the Unit 1 explosion, the fallout arrived over Hawaii. On or about the sixth day after the Unit 1 explosion, the fallout was expected to arrive on the west coast of North America. On or about the 10th day (~March 22nd), the initial plume of fallout should have arrived over the eastern half of the United States. To summarize, I estimate that the fallout from the first plume hit:

- Hawaii on March 15th
- The west coast of North America by March 18th
- Central parts of North America by March 20th
- The east coast of North America by March 22nd

Then if we consider the last most intense release from Fukushima for the month of March, that latter plume would likely have arrived over North America's east coast by April 3rd or 4th. To understand where the fallout may have landed, we need to understand whether or not these time lines coincided with local rainstorm activity.

Chart 2.3, National Weather Service: California Precipitation for March 16th - 22nd illustrates the cumulative rain fall over California at exactly the optimal time to insure high titers of radioactivity would befall most of California from the first plume arriving from Fukushima.[204]

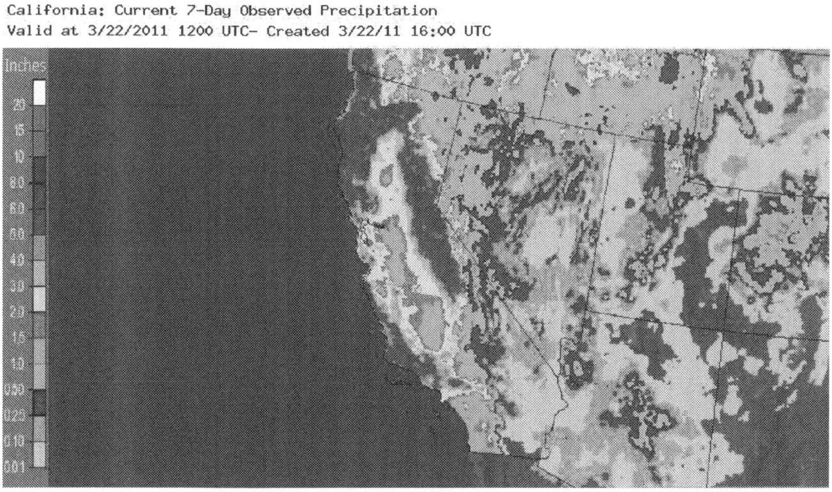
California: Current 7-Day Observed Precipitation
Valid at 3/22/2011 1200 UTC- Created 3/22/11 16:00 UTC
Inches

Chart 2.3 Cal. Precipitation for March 16th through 22nd, 2011
Source: National Weather Service

Yet mysteriously, Chart 2.2 above does not reflect the massive, expected landfall of fallout during this time period (March 16th - March 22nd). How could this be, by design or by default?

We simply do not know. We may speculate it could have been either. But what is established is that the technology used to monitor radiation levels by the EPA had (and continues to have) ongoing performance gaps at numerous regional monitoring stations.[205] Such performance gaps and shut down monitoring equipment should explain why radiation levels defied detection at critical potential hot spots across the United States. What we have in the midst of such shoddy science is the EPA's own records that depict spikes over the greater Sacramento area as follows:

- ✓ ~March 18th
- ✓ ~April 1st
- ✓ ~ April 6th
- ✓ ~April 9th

- ✓ ~April 14th-16th
- ✓ ~April 23rd
- ✓ ~April 25th-May 17th
- ✓ ~May 23rd
- ✓ ~June 3rd
- ✓ ~June 7th
- ✓ ~June 13th-June 21st
- ✓ ~July 2nd-6th

Rainstorms such as the ones appearing above California traveled across most of the United States during the aforementioned critical times. For example, beginning April 4th, a series of rainstorms that pounded the southeastern United States was again recorded by the National Weather Service. These storms were traveling over 800 miles per day. They were likely transporting vast amounts of radioactive fallout arising from the last plume out of Fukushima just ten days prior during the month of March.[206]

It appears that we might not be able to completely rely on official United States data gathering for air measurements. Recently, the Washington State Department of Health announced it would be taking air samples via a specially equipped helicopter to ascertain real-time fallout levels above the greater Seattle region. But they also stated that because of "national security concerns," they intend to selectively withhold that data from the public's eye.[207]

In the meantime, if we wish to make an attempt to further appraise the devastating fallout in light of possibly skewed data, we may turn to the record amounts of radiation that fell upon select regions of our United States water shed, as well as to reported amounts that appeared in United States milk supplies.[208, 209, 210]

Radiation in the Oceans

The radioactive contamination that has now entered the surrounding ocean is at least 10 times (i.e., at least one order of magnitude) higher than that released from the Chernobyl Catastrophe over similar expanses of water.[211] According to the Woods Hole Oceanographic Institute's chart below (which was compiled pre-Fukushima), a rough estimate would be to simply multiply the below figures (by at least seven times) pertaining to the Northern Pacific Ocean by 2014.[212]

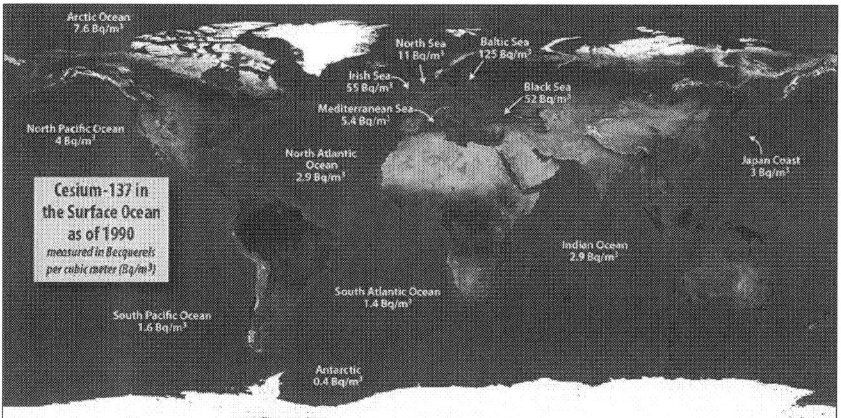

Chart 2.4 Cesium-137 in the Oceans, 1990
Source: Woods Hole Oceanographic Institute

According to oceanic currents shown in Chart 2.5, Hawaii could expect radioactive ocean currents to wash up on its shore by March 2012, and from there onto the North American west coast by no later than 2014.[213,214]

However, along the southern California oceanic ecosystems it is now known that radiation levels for radioactive sulfur spiked 2.5 times above average levels by March 28th, 2011, due to Jet Stream delivery of Fukushima fallout.[215] Additionally the Jet Stream was also responsible for delivering radioactive iodine into the marine ecosystem off of Vancouver, Canada. For example, seaweeds off the coast there accumulated radioactive iodine to the tune of 400% over safety standards.[216] Over time, all subsequent fallout contributions by the Jet Stream will only compound the slower ocean current delivery of radionuclides into the bioaccumulation process, significantly increasing health risks from consuming North American seafood from the west coast.

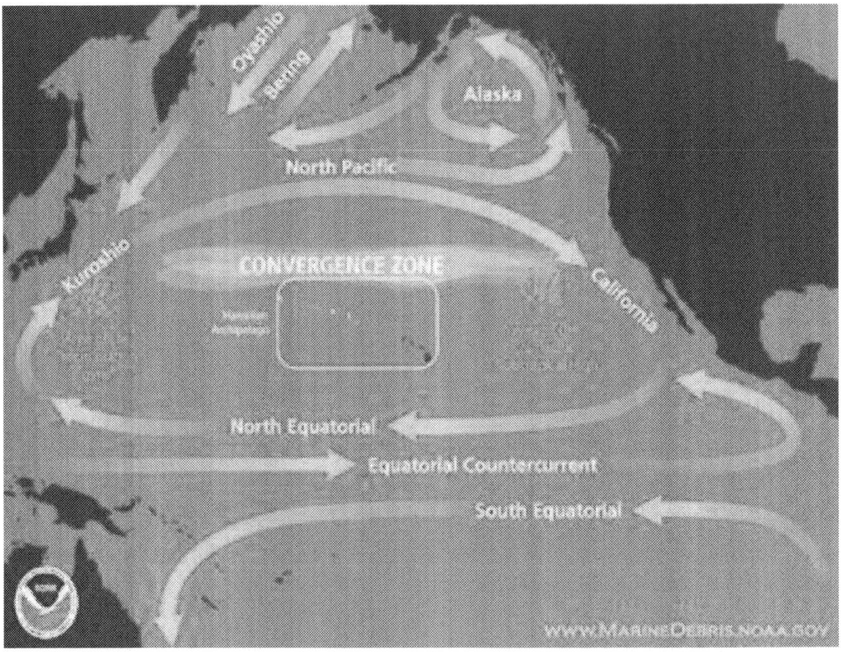

Chart 2.5 Ocean Currents
Source: National Oceanic and Atmospheric Administration

The Pacific Ocean is one of the top food sources for people living on its coastlines. The western one-third of the Northern Pacific Ocean corridor nearest to Japan must now be considered contaminated. The middle one-third is likely to be contaminated by mid-2012. The final one-third hugging the west coast of North America will likely be highly contaminated by 2014.

Chart 2.6 shows a satellite image from 160 kilometers (100 miles) north of the Fukushima nuclear power plant in Japan. Japan's two large ocean currents - the Kuroshio and the Oyashio - converge here.

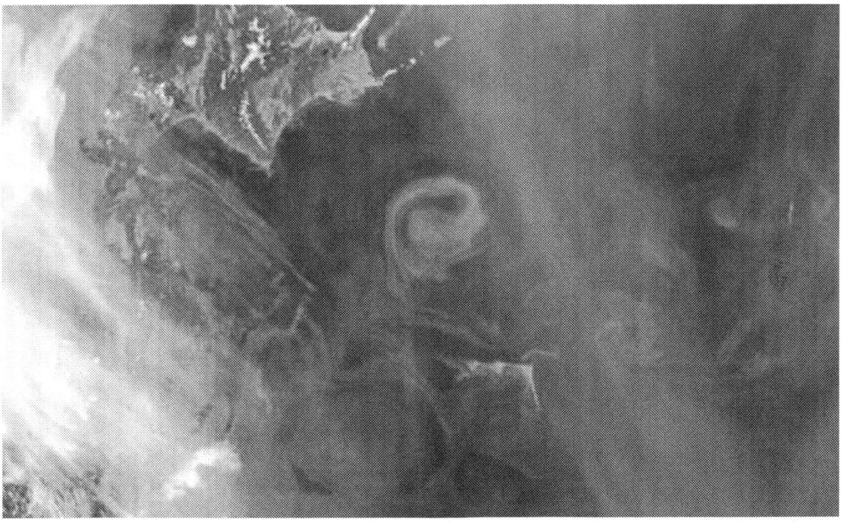

Chart 2.6 Ocean Currents North of Fukushima
Source: NASA

For more information, visit the website dedicated to providing complete simulation up-to-dates of the Fukushima Catastrophe.[217]

Potential Radiation Doses Post Fukushima

As of August 2011, the Fukushima radioactivity left the air and entered into the soils and watersheds across the globe. Simultaneously, we saw continuous ongoing releases from the stricken Fukushima Daiichi Nuclear Power Plant. For example, on March 15th TEPCO reported that the releases from the nuclear power plant skyrocketed up to 2,000 Trillion Bq/hour (0.002 X 10^{15}Bq/hr).

From that point forward into early April, it appears that 137Cs (which easily becomes an aerosol during violent nuclear accidents) spewed most heavily across the Pacific Ocean onto North American soils. In many locations across North America, fallout exceeded that deposited onto many parts of the Japanese soils to the north and south from "ground zero" of the accident. For example, by April 6th, 2011, the official French atmospheric monitoring agency Centre d'Enseignement et de Recherche en Environnement Atmosphrique (or CEREA) used the best available data to simulate the fallout pattern provided in the chart below. Other official public monitoring agencies from Norway, Germany and Austria showed similar tracing amounts in their simulations as well:[218, 219]

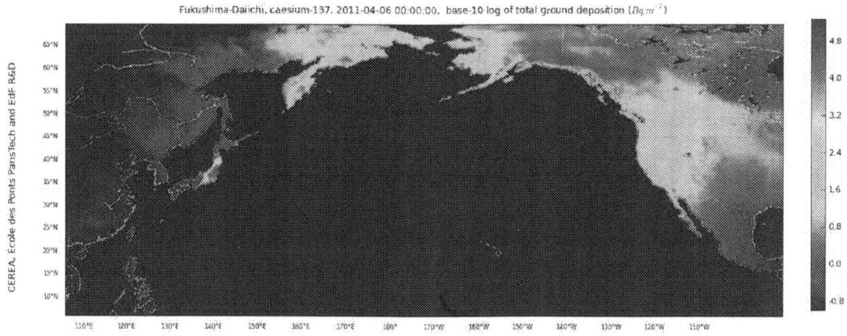

Chart 2.7 Distribution of Cesuim-137 as of July 19, 2011
Source: Centre d'Enseignement et de Recherche en Environnement Atmosphérique

By July 19th, 2011, the releases at Fukushima Daiichi Nuclear Power Plant continued, averaging 1 Billion Bq/hour.[220]

Japan's Environment Ministry released their survey on 137Cs on August 29th, 2011. Their report covered 469 incinerator operators from 16 prefectures in Tohoku and Kanto from late June into August. High levels of 137Cs were recorded in dust at 42 incineration plants in seven of these prefectures, including Chiba and Iwate. The report revealed that the highest 137Cs levels in the dust ranged from 95,300 Bq/kilogram in Fukushima Prefecture, 70,800 Bq/kilogram in Chiba Prefecture, and 30,000 Bq/kilogram in Iwate Prefecture. Chillingly, even the lower levels determined at other incinerators exceeded 8,000 Bq/kilogram in Ibaraki, Tochigi, Gunma and Tokyo.[221]

All of these Bq/kilogram "convert" into "roentgen equivalent man" (rem) or millirems when these radioactive particles contaminate a human with direct skin contact, by inhalation or by ingestion. Due to direct exposure and a process discussed later called bioaccumulation, even minor levels of Bq/kilogram in the biosphere will rapidly build up within us harmful levels of millirems. The build-up continues to increase the longer we dwell in contaminated regions. For example, it only takes a few hundred millirems per person to cause significant cancer throughout a given population.

Alarmingly, zones in Japan where folks are now living (but located just outside of the government's too unsafe to live "exclusion zone") have been found with lethal levels of 137Cs scattered over wide territories.

According to Japan's Ministry of Education, Culture, Sports, Science and Technology (MEXT), among the highest recorded dose levels cumulative over five months are: (50,810 mrem) at Koirino, Okuma-cho, (22,370 mrem) at both Kawafusa and Namie-cho, (17,240 mrem) at Futaba-cho, (11,530 mrem) at both Koryougahama and Tomioka-cho, and (5,310 mrem) at Kanaya, Kotaka-ku and Minamisouma-shi.[222]

In the United States, the Federal agencies responsible for protecting us from radioactive exposures enforce regulations stating that the dose limit shall not exceed 100 millirems (100 mrem) per year, per person.[223] The EPA advises that approximately one-third of this amount (~200 mrem/yr arising from radon alone) is responsible for thousands of cancer deaths each year.[224] As the Director of the Institute for Energy and Environmental Research (IEER), Dr. Arjun Makhijani, comments, "... Using the 2006 National Academies risk estimates for cancer, 620 millirem per year to each of the 311 million people in the United States would eventually be associated with about 200,000 cancers each year, about half of them fatal."[225,226,227]

Well, here are the facts! Before the Fukushima Catastrophe, on average, a person living in America received 360 mrem/yr![228] Therefore, according to the statistical methods published by the National Academy of Sciences referenced above, average annual United States radiation exposure is responsible for at least 100,000 cancers each year, with half of these expected to be lethal. Any other additional radiation exposure obviously dramatically increases our cancer rates.

Here in North America, Fukushima fallout during rainstorms continued to be at dangerous levels into late summer 2011. One YouTube amateur video documented Geiger counter readings from rain collected on July 18th, 2011 in the surrounding Vancouver regions in British Columbia. The video clearly shows that the readings jumped to 1.66 microSv/hour – a reading that "officially" mandates immediate evacuation from the area.[229] If this dose were to hold constant for an entire year, it would exceed the permissible annual dose by 1,450% (~1,450 mrem/year). Then, the collective rainfall doses would creep insidiously into the food chain.

And now we have one EPA chart revealing devastating spikes arriving onto U.S. soils, suggesting ongoing, uncontrolled chain reactions were still occurring at Fukushima Daiichi Nuclear Power Plant almost six months later.[230]

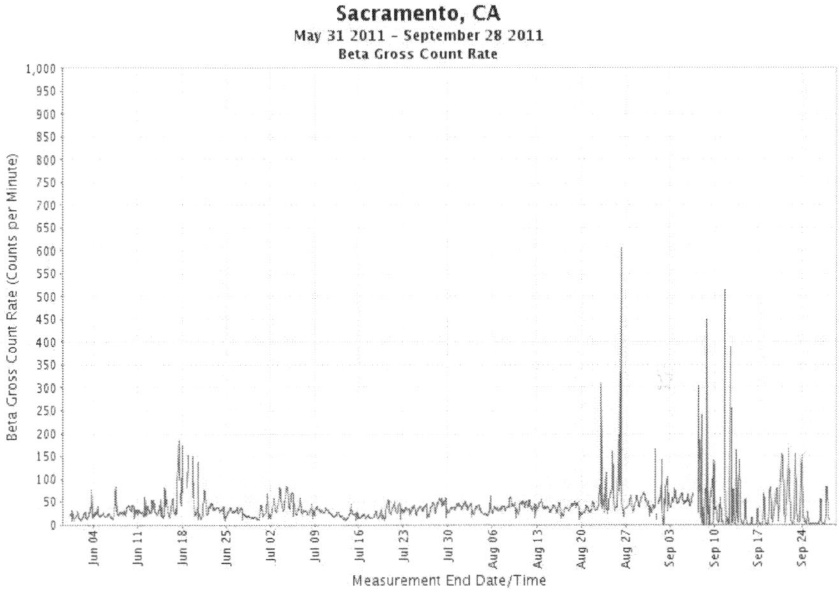

Chart 2.8 Radiation in Sacramento MAY 31 through September 28, 2011
Source: Environmental Protection Agency (EPA)

Therefore, it is only prudent to take all appropriate measures to protect ourselves and our children from this latest nuclear age crisis crossing the Pacific and circulating around the world. I have specifically written *Fukushima Meltdown & Modern Radiation* to enable many of you to easily accomplish this crucial goal.

Radiation in Drinking Water

The EPA sets the Maximum Contaminant Level (MCL) of radiation in our drinking water originating from 131-I alone to be 3 pico Curies per liter (3 pCi/L).[231]

Normally the rainwater in Boise, ID runs radiation levels at 0.2 pCi/L. But well after expected arrival of Fukushima Fallout on March 22nd, that level skyrocketed to 242 pCi/L, and then as the second wave hit, it soared as high as 390 pCi/L on March 27th or 130 times over EPA permissible levels! More specifically in early April, the EPA recorded that the 134Cs content (half-life of two years, but with a biological impact lasting over 20 years) rose by over 13 times normal levels in Boise (up to 41 pCi/L). With a half-life of 30 years, but with a biological impact lasting more than 300 years, 137Cs was found to rise by 12 times more than normal levels (up to 36 pCi/L). Boise can expect to have water shed issues for many decades ahead.

Here is information on other cities where the data was captured by the EPA for 131-I (in alphabetical order):

- Boston, MA (collected March 22nd) ➔ 92 pCi/L or 30 times over EPA permissible levels
- Jacksonville, FL (collected March 31st) ➔ 150 pCi/L or 50 times over EPA permissible level
- Montgomery, Alabama (collected March 30th) ➔ 3.7 pCi/L
- Olympia, WA (collected March 24th) ➔ 125 pCi/L or 41 times over EPA permissible level
- Portland, OR (collected March 25th) ➔ 86.8 pCi/L or 28 times over EPA permissible level

- Richmond, CA (collected March 22nd) ➔ 138 pCi/L or 46 times over EPA permissible level
- Salt Lake City, UT (collected March 17th) ➔ 8.1 pCi/L[232]

At one point on March 23rd (collected from 9AM to 6PM PDT), the rainwater in San Francisco exceeded the permissible EPA's drinking water limits by 18,100% as it rose to 543 pCi/L.[233, 234]

United States Milk Supply Contamination

More disturbing is trying to determine the level of radiation being ingested by our children. Milk in Hawaii was discovered on April 4th, 2011 to contain 18 pCi/L of 131-I, 24 pCi/L of 134Cs and 19 pCi/L of 137Cs. Radiation in our bodies is cumulative, so these amounts are simply devastating to the health of all who consume the milk. Considering the half-life of the latter two radionuclides, unless aggressive remediation measures are taken to remove these contaminants from the food chain of these dairy herds, there will be decades-long consequences, just like there has been in the greater Chernobyl regions.[235, 236]

On March 30th radiation in milk supplies in Little Rock, AK was recorded to be 8.9 pCi/L for 131-I, and later that same week, Phoenix, AR reported 3.2 pCi/L and Los Angeles, CA 2.9 pCi/L for 131-I.

The Department of Nuclear Engineering at Berkeley is maintaining up-to-date tracking of several radionuclides in milk samples for the greater San Francisco Bay area. Although Berkeley is downplaying the levels currently found in the samples, they fail to state that all internally absorbed radionuclides become a greater and greater cumulative health threat, since these radioactive particles are retained for extended time periods. Children will be especially impacted in this regard, and all the more so as the expected 90Sr enters into the U.S. milk supply.[237, 238]

Now, here is the catch - the derived intervention levels or DIL (sounds official, right?) determined by the Food and Drug Administration (FDA) states that the permissible radiation levels in milk is 1,500 times greater than that permissible for our drinking water. Who would have guessed? So, should we all rest assured that our kids remain safe and sound if they prefer milk over water, even though the National Research Council and other ethically-minded official agencies have repeatedly stated there are no safe levels of radiation for human beings?[239, 240] I find myself wondering who were the medical doctors and radiation biologists that created these standards?

We can all be sure of one thing - the regions that have had these high radiation readings in milk, water and food supplies will bioaccumulate[241] the radioactive hazardous materials for decades to come, insuring continuous risk to our children.

Radioactivity Released by Fukushima

Some of the radioactive particles that vaporized during the detonation explosion have been arriving on the west coast of the United States and Canada affecting the air we breathe. Assuming that North America is receiving the same kinds of radioactive fallout as it did during the Chernobyl crisis of 1986, since March 18th, 2011, United States has sequentially received health destroying levels of:[242]

- ✓ Barium-140 (140Ba)
- ✓ Beryllium-7 (7Be)
- ✓ Cerium-141 (141Ce)

- ✓ Cerium-144 (144Ce)
- ✓ Cesium-134 (134Cs)
- ✓ Cesium-136 (136Cs)
- ✓ Cesium-137 (137Cs)
- ✓ Cobalt-60 (60Co)
- ✓ Curium-242 (242Cm)
- ✓ Fe (Iron)-59 (59Fe)
- ✓ Iodine-131 (131-I)
- ✓ Iodine-132 (132-I)
- ✓ Lanthanum-140 (140La)
- ✓ Molybdenum-95 (95Mb)
- ✓ Manganese-54 (54Mn)
- ✓ Neptunium-239 (239Np)
- ✓ Niobium-95 (95Nb)
- ✓ Plutonium-238 (238Pu)
- ✓ Plutonium-239 (239Pu)
- ✓ Plutonium-240 (240Pu)
- ✓ Plutonium-241 (241Pu)
- ✓ Ruthenium-103 (103Ru)
- ✓ Ruthenium-106 (106Ru)
- ✓ Strontium-89 (89Sr)
- ✓ Strontium-90 (90Sr)

- ✓ Tellurium-132 (132Te)
- ✓ Xenon-33 (33Xe)
- ✓ Zinc-65 (65Zn)
- ✓ Zirconium-95 (95Zr)

Perhaps just as importantly, the Chernobyl releases of radiation, and their bioaccumulation impact, continued well past the next decade following the catastrophe.[243, 244, 245, 246, 247] Yet the health impact here in North America from the Chernobyl Catastrophe's releases of radionuclides, including escalations in infant mortality, thyroid cancer, breast cancer and AIDS, has never been fully disclosed to the American people.[248, 249, 250, 251, 252]

It is also highly probable that the Chernobyl incident released significant amounts of Chloride-36 (half-life = 30,000 years), Technetium-99 (half-life = 211,000 years), plus Xenon-137, and one uranium daughter product Iodine-129. But don't hold your breath expecting government officials to give us all the details in a timely manner regarding what has landed on North America from the Fukushima disaster of March 2011, even though there is significant corroborating data. Instead the U.S. Environmental Protection Agency (EPA) and Health Canada have reduced or shut down government monitoring claiming that it is not necessary because no significant radioactivity has reached North America.[253, 254] Independent data has proven otherwise.

As of May 12, 2011, there is absolute certainty that North America has received the following radioactive elements from the Fukushima Daiichi Nuclear Power Plant fallout:[255, 256, 257, 258, 259, 260]

Cesium-134 and 137 (134Cs & 137Cs). Radioactive cesium appears closely associated with increased risk for primary invalidism, blood disorders, cardiac arrhythmias, autoimmune diseases (i.e., thyroiditis, diabetes), severe debilitating neuromuscular disease, reproductive abnormalities and cancer (especially thyroid cancer, breast cancer, liver cancer and leukemia).[261, 262] It easily replaces essential potassium reserves inside cells while oxidizing internal cell proteins and fats.

Iodine-131 (131-I). 131-I is known to cause thyroid cancer and severe impairment of the immune system, especially in the young, the old, and in the immune compromised population.[263]

Plutonium-238 and 239 (238Pu & 239Pu). Radioactive plutonium appears closely associated with cardiovascular disease, leukemia, lung cancer, breast cancer, several childhood cancers, infant mortality and trans-generational mutations.[264]

Strontium-89 and 90 (89Sr & 90Sr). Radioactive strontium is known to cause bone cancer and severe bone deformities.[265]

Uranium-234 and 238 (234U & 238U). Radioactive uranium places those exposed at high risk for cancer, miscarriages, still births, childhood cancers, birth defects, infertility, severe or crippling brain disorders including crippling childhood developmental disorders or kidney disease. In addition, both 234U and 238U induce genetic abnormalities long term.[266]

The Nature and Dangers of Radioactive Elements

There are no safe levels of radiation, no matter what some officials claim to the contrary.[267] There are specific radioactive fission and decay "daughter" products that all arise from the "parent" radioactive element uranium. Uranium is the key fuel to nuclear reactors.[268] These daughter radionuclides either decay over time into new elements that may also be radioactive, or they may remain the same element but with less radioactive energy.[269] This is called the decay chain. A daughter radionuclide may decay into an entirely different radionuclide (called transmutation). The decay rate of any given radionuclide has, on average, a certain half-life. The half-life is defined as the amount of time it takes, on average, for one half of the radionuclide to decay.[270]

As the decay chain rolls out over time, the new half-life of the next daughter radionuclide can either be greater than or less than the half-life of the "parent" radionuclide. The half-life is only a mathematical trend, not an exact timetable of decay.[271] Also, the daughter radionuclide can possess greater ionizing energy than the parent, such as Strontium-90 decaying and transmuting into Yittrium-90.[272] Therefore, a mixture of radionuclides falling onto any given region (a so called "hot spot") may result in a much more deadly "ionizing footprint" than that suspected from the half-life of any one radionuclide alone. Beyond this, the ionizing footprint of destruction may continue well past any particle's respective half-life, by at least three times, and even up to 10 times longer.[273]

During the initial 12 days of a nuclear accident, three of the most prominent and dangerous particles that may have easily travelled around the globe via the Jet Stream and then released in rainfall fallout to the ground are 131-I, 137Cs and 140Ba. Going into the second and third years, the evolution of the decay products becomes more and more dominated by 141Ce, 95Zr and 89Sr. During the coming years, the predominant decay products will become more and more dominated by bone destroying 90Sr and cell destroying 137Cs as others decay away.[274] From that point forward, 90Sr and 137Cs continue to impact the food chain and all associated life forms for many decades, raining down, so to speak, untold horrors because it is difficult to track where they may fall out or may have already fallen out and deposited in the environment. In the case of the Fukushima Catastrophe, it appears that significant amounts of the lung-destroying 239Pu and other radioactive isotopes were ejected.

Recently, the teeth from children known to have been exposed to radioactive fallout have been shown to collect 90Sr.[275] Collecting childhood teeth after they normally fall out can serve as a perfect record to accurately track this horror. As a result of this new tracking system, it is now clear that the Petkau Effect and regional "hot spot" bioaccumulation of radionuclides into the food chain are far more devastating to those living in Japan than the scientific establishment has been willing to admit. They use the industry promoted linear models that ignore radiation behaviors in biological systems.[276]

I estimate that the devastating health impact upon North Americans during the next several decades will actually be many multiples of any predictions that will be forecasted by the scientific establishment. The four key radionuclides that people should keep a close eye on will be 131-I, 137Cs, 90Sr and 239Pu. Later in *Fukushima Meltdown & Modern Radiation: Protecting Ourselves and our Future Generations* I will share: (a) expected time frames for the waves of illnesses to arrive, (b) their likely duration, as well as the (c) specific kinds of illnesses that may result.

Measuring the Spread of Radioactive Fallout

The first method for determining the total release in comparison to Chernobyl is to consider that the releases at Fukushima will be ongoing for many months and possibly years to come.[277, 278] This comes from the initial explosions, the ongoing steam vapor releases, the ongoing water table contamination, the dumping of radioactive water into the ocean, the multiple criticalities (chain reactions) that spewed radioactivity invisibly and repeatedly into the atmosphere, and finally the bioaccumulation and biomagnification of this new burden of radioactivity into the regional and global food chain.

We briefly mentioned above the IRSN and ZAMG collection and collating of radiation fallout data around the Pacific's Ring of Fire region covering March 12th - 22nd. The following is a forensic analysis of those tallies that supports my projections for the scale of the Fukushima Catastrophe, plus plausible scenarios that sooner or later will only add to the catastrophe. For the sake of simplicity, we will focus our discussion on only one radionuclide, 137Cs, due to its ability to bioaccumulate, hide in the biosphere of hundreds of years, and damage the health of our children and families for many generations.

At least 75% of the fuel rods have been damaged at Units 1 through 3 at Fukushima Daiichi Nuclear Power Plant,[279] so how much 137Cs went air-borne at the time of the explosions and fires at Units 1 through 4 verses how much went into steam, into the water table or into the ocean? And how much of the undamaged fuel remains? Japanese scientists claim that 99% of the cesium remains trapped in the water; however, data in US Nuclear Regulatory Standards indicates that no cesium will be retained in boiling water, and that is exactly the condition that existed at Fukushima.

On March 21st, 2011, a secret report delivered at a Stanford University forum by Areva, perhaps the largest nuclear power conglomerate in Europe, stated that it was likely that the earthquake of March 11th enabled the core temperatures in Units 1, 2 and 3 to reach approximately 2,000°C for at least seven hours each. Furthermore, Areva reported that up to 75%

of the nuclear fuel rods in each of these units were exposed to such temperatures for seven hours or longer.[280] We now know that all three reactor vessel containments were breached, thus allowing vast amounts of radiation to spike intermittently, and slowly leak out into the local, regional and eventually global biosphere.[281]

Initially, there was both an explosion as well as fires at the Unit 4 storage fuel pool. We know that the pool remained largely intact from those initial explosions. But as of May 13th, 2011, the Unit 4 building (which housed the storage fuel pool) was structurally so unstable that the risk of collapse grew daily.[282] If the entire building collapsed, then the storage fuel pool was also likely to rapidly drain, thereby exposing the majority of the remaining undamaged spent fuel rods to open air. Should that happen, the portion of the fuel rods exposed to air would rapidly begin to melt. If the fuel rods could not be kept cool with water, meltdown temperatures would soon reach over 2,000°C. Once the temperatures of these fuel rods approached 2,000°C, it would only be a matter of a few hours for the remaining potential radiation stores to be released broadly into the open environment.

If the Unit 4 building did collapse during an aftershock, it would likely render uninhabitable the northern half of Japan for an extended period, should the wind blow in "the wrong direction." If volunteer teams remained onsite in an attempt to keep the fuel rods in the collapsed building sprayed with sufficient fresh water, they would be working against the odds that the sprays could even reach the fuel rods with so much of the building collapsed on top of the draining/ drained fuel pool. Regardless, over time due to the lack of containment, the entire load of 137Cs (1560 Kilograms - an Apocalyptic amount) would escape to the local, regional and global biosphere.

There is a mammoth common storage spent fuel pool that was used by all the reactors and was located in close proximity to the Unit 4 building that remained stable. This storage unit contained 6,375 spent fuel assemblies. Of these assemblies, the ones less than 30-years-old would likely have the highest percentages of 137Cs of all the fuel rods at the facility.[283] Therefore, if the Unit 4 building collapsed, an evacuation would be ordered requiring workers to leave. With no one to maintain adequate coolant in this mammoth shared storage fuel pool, the world would face a global game changer of Biblical proportions. On July 9th, a 7.1 magnitude aftershock again rocked the Fukushima Daiichi nuclear power plant necessitating yet another evacuation of the Fukushima crews who were managing the coolant systems. Fortunately this time around, the threat subsided without further damage to any onsite facility.[284]

From this sets of facts, it was prophetic for the Executive Vice President of Areva, Dr. Matthias Braun, to state, "Clearly, we are witnessing one of the greatest disasters in modern times."[285] But even more definitively (as if it were even possible), a top nuclear operations expert, Arnie Gundersen, stated flat out that, "Fukushima is the biggest industrial catastrophe in the history of mankind."[286]

The Human Impact of the Fukushima Catastrophe

Many scientists have concluded that the Japanese people were lucky during the initial explosions that rocked Fukushima Daiichi Nuclear Power Plant because the prevailing wind currents blew the largest portions of the highly toxic radioactivity out toward the sea rather than inland. These scientists believe (or state for the record so that we believe) that the ocean will simply dilute the radiation's lethality down next to nothing. This is incorrect. Airborne 137Cs and 134Cs from the Fukushima accident was detected in milk as far away as Vermont in April and May, clearly indicating that the 137Cs was in the process of entering the world's food chain.[287, 288]

Horrifyingly, according to data compiled by the Environmental Protection Agency (EPA) and the Centers for Disease Control and Prevention (CDC), since March 17th, there is compelling evidence that the infant death rate average from four United States west coast states (Washington, Oregon, Idaho and California) jumped 35%.[289] Respectively, children, infants and fetuses are from 10 to thousands of times more susceptible to radiation poisoning than healthy adults, as are the very old and those with immune deficiency syndromes.[290] Other parts of the United States will also follow this trend.

For another chilling example, parts of Pennsylvania during the initial stages of the Fukushima Catastrophe received the highest level of rainfall in the United States. Recall that rain brings fallout down to the earth. Coincidently, the areas hardest hit by this rainfall (in the greater Philadelphia region) experienced a 48% increase in infant mortality rates according to CDC data, much higher than along the United States west coast for the same time period! In a June 17th interview with Shawnette Wilson on June Fox News 29 at 10PM, Joseph Mangano, Executive Director of the Radiation and Public Health Project, reported on this unexplained rise in infant deaths.[291] Due to the stir the segment caused, Fox News took the video down from its MyFoxPhilly.com website, and the segment was posted to YouTube.[292] As you can infer, this trend in higher infant mortality rates is expected to worsen over the next year or more given the historical experiences from Chernobyl.

On July 11th, 2001, there was a stunning report in the Vancouver Sun concerning a joint news conference with the

Ministry of Public Safety and Solicitor General and the B.C. Coroners Service, which confirmed that for the first six months of 2011, the infant mortality rate spiked nearly 60% over the previous year (21 infant deaths from January until the end of June, verses a grand total of 16 for the entire year of 2010).[293] Will we now see these dramatic escalations in North America's infant death rates play out in all three areas by the first anniversary of the Fukushima Catastrophe?

Due to many factors (one of which is the slow process of bioaccumulation that hoards larger and larger amounts of radiation right up the food chain and the other being the long half-life of many radionuclides in fallout),[294, 295] the net number of expected human cancers will trend upward, not downward.[296] So, let us ask ourselves one simple question…

> *If in terms of raw radioactivity, the Fukushima Catastrophe is seven to 42 times the Chernobyl Catastrophe (depending upon multiple of radiation released or the impact upon the multiple of radiation released coupled to a six-fold higher regional population), what human death toll may we expect during the next 20 years?*

The chilling answer to that question may have been provided in a recent publication by the New York Academy of Sciences that utilized more than 5,000 authoritative Russian publications to draw some startling conclusions. The Russian investigators have updated the mortality rates from the Chernobyl incident to at least 985,000 and linked no less than 8,000,000 serious injuries and cases of severe chronic diseases to this single event.[297]

Unfortunately it took at least 20 years before scientists and medical doctors could tabulate enough factual data to gauge the Chernobyl Catastrophe's devastating impact. However, this timeline offers us a template with which to forecast the human death toll and disabling injuries that may manifest from the Fukushima Catastrophe by 2031. In making these critical projections, the next 20 years are the first timeline of concern, and the following 80 years are the second timeline of concern.

Assuming the above rates of morbidity and mortality for the Chernobyl Catastrophe are correct, follow-on projections from the Fukushima Catastrophe will likely fall somewhere between 7 times to 42 times these figures. I have examined many of the mathematical models scientific experts utilize to estimate future projections of deaths and serious debilitating injuries from radiation accidents. I was specifically struck by the data on historical morbidity and mortality rates relating to bioaccumulation of toxins into the food chain.

Bioaccumulations of radionuclides from nuclear power plant catastrophes such as the Chernobyl incident may accrue into inland human populations by a factor of 10 to 100 times that of the soil contamination.[298] In the case of radionuclides polluting great bodies of water, by volume the biomagnification up the food chain and into mammal tissues could add up to 300 times that originally found in the water.[299] So, even as the environmental (soil, air and water) concentrations of radioactivity are reported as lessening in any given region, the food chain accumulation has the potential to more than make up for this apparent environmental loss proving that in examining radioactivity, we must look at the entire biosphere and not allow the data to be cherry-picked.

Some Chilling Conclusions

I think we can rationally conclude that the Fukushima Catastrophe will result in much greater mortality and morbidity rates than the Chernobyl Catastrophe, as exhaustively tabulated by Yablokov et al.[300]

Consider the facts I have presented so far:

- ✓ ZAMG's 137Cs data provided compelling evidence the Fukushima Catastrophe was spewing out fallout equivalent to one Chernobyl Catastrophe every four to 20 days.
- ✓ Hirsch presented data calculated from impeccable authorities showing that the amount of 131-I and 137Cs released from the Fukushima Catastrophe was already on the scale of three Chernobyl Catastrophes as early as March 23rd, 2011.
- ✓ Bowyer's 33Xe data indicated that as of March 28th, 2011 the Fukushima Catastrophe released approximately two to five times the amount of radiation than the Chernobyl Catastrophe.
- ✓ Woods Hole data documented that by May 18th, 2011, the Fukushima accident released 10 times more radiation into the ocean than was released during the Chernobyl Catastrophe.
- ✓ Bioaccumulation and biomagnification are known to amplify radiation exposure for humans from 10 to 300 times the original radiation release into the local and regional biosphere.
- ✓ The fallout from Fukushima skyrocketed twice as high into the air as the Chernobyl Fallout.
- ✓ The calculations given in Table 2.1 above concerning the likely extent of the damaged Daiichi fuel rods

estimates the damage to be no less than seven times greater than the Chernobyl Catastrophe.

Collectively, these chilling reports give us even greater pause when we consider that the US will continue to receive additional fallout from the Fukushima accident for months down the road. Taken altogether, Arnie Gundersen has uniquely and correctly characterized the Fukushima tragedy as a "Chernobyl on Steroids."[301]

In fact, rarely have prospective environmental or projected human health impact studies based upon the internationally recognized mathematical models designed to accurately assess radiation accidents ever come close to what actually does occur.[302] For example, the gold standard for dose, dose limits and health risks originated with the International Commission on Radiological Protection (ICRP). This gold standard is based upon a model concept of an "equivalent dose" of radiation thought to be present in a given circumstance. To then become biologically meaningful, the equivalent dose is converted into an "effective dose" relating to its impact upon the cells, tissues, organs and whole body. This gold standard has been designed to accurately forecast in advance the best estimates on the health risks to those exposed. But this gold standard forecasting model was never designed to incorporate actual nuclear accident consequences of the past which give us real, actual, historical mortality and morbidity rates of any given exposed individual, group or population. It is merely a theoretical model system that has rarely, if ever, gotten it right.[303,304,305,306]

Common sense tells me we should reconsider such "gold standards" and stick to the most historically accurate numbers determined via exhaustive retrospective analysis and then reconcile all the common denominators to derive the most reliable forecast. With all the spin, under reporting and misreporting common to radiation environmental impact studies dominated by special interests, this is not easily done.[307] The special interests are essentially pulling the strings of Federal agencies ensuring they promote the science of doubt instead of the science of common sense. In other words, the "bending of science" has never been greater than the historical M.O. of official national and international radiation monitoring agencies. This latest crisis at Fukushima has driven this point home once again.[308, 309, 310, 311, 312, 313, 314, 315]

Therefore, to deal with our current exposure problems, I have spent considerable time qualifying all my data sources. I based my mathematical forecasts only on exhaustive retrospective studies,[316, 317, 318, 319, 320] plus real historical biomarkers[321, 322] that clearly share the best common denominators inherent to the Fukushima Catastrophe. I believe the brunt of the transgenerational impact on the world-wide human population will only be fully realized over several hundreds of years, but especially during the first 100 years. Therefore, I chose to break down this next 100 years into two separate time periods because since 1953 we now have several very accurate, well-defined, historical health assessment time periods covering multiple fallout events.[323, 324, 325, 326, 327]

During the next 20 years my calculations show that approximately 7,000,000 human beings scattered across the globe will die as a direct result of the 2011 Fukushima Catastrophe, and approximately 64,000,000 will be plagued by debilitating radiation induced chronic illnesses, unless they learn some of the unique ways to protect themselves. I outline protection measures in Parts II and III of *Fukushima Meltdown & Modern Radiation: Protecting Ourselves and our Future Generations.*

Second, due to the associated half-lives of these lethal toxins, my calculations also show that during the following 80 years, another 7,000,000 will die and another 64,000,000 will contract serious radiation induced illnesses as a direct result of the 2011 Fukushima Catastrophe. Both these projections would include escalations in fetus deaths, as well as congenital deformities and disabilities.[328, 329]

These predictions translate into 14 times the current morbidity and mortality rates due to the Chernobyl Catastrophe. However, additional containment failure or escalations in current leakage pathways or subsequent major radioactive releases would dramatically influence upward any forecasts.

Finally, after careful consideration and review of the best current and historical epidemiological data, I estimate that from 5% to 15% of the total mortality and morbidity figures above will apply specifically to North America over the next 100 years.

Surely my forecasts will stir a great debate. But in the end (and provided we take an honest and unprecedented global undertaking to properly appraise mortality and morbidity rates as best exemplified to date by Yablokov et al.), only history will reveal the true extent of the horrors caused by this latest nuclear catastrophe.

Part II

Protecting Your Family

Many people are asking what they can do to protect themselves and their families from the Fukushima Daiichi radioactive fallout. Since the 1950's, Americans have been suffering from the fallout of above ground nuclear bomb testing, and the opening of more than 100 hundred nuclear power facilities and weapons plants across the United States. This combination of accelerated fallout and constant exposure to low-level radioactivity is compromising human health throughout the U.S. Canadians face equally serious exposures as the British Columbia data points out. My purpose in writing *Fukushima Meltdown & Modern Radiation: Protecting Ourselves and our Future Generations* is to help people find solutions to regenerating their health on an ongoing basis.

Human physiology is simply not well designed to handle even the lowest doses of radiation without injury to our cells, tissues and organs, including our immune systems. This is especially true for the very young and the very old. In the very young, not enough time has elapsed for innate resistance to fully mature. In the very old, the exposure to radiation from all sources accumulates over time. The body burden of radionuclides and exposure to radiation during a person's lifetime amplifies the aging process and contributes greatly to the development of chronic degenerative disease. Although it remains controversial, it certainly does appear that radiation exposures increase the likelihood of sustained genetic abnormalities that are passed down for many generations.[330, 331, 332, 333, 334, 335, 336]

For most of you reading *Fukushima Meltdown & Modern Radiation*, you know that we have few options when it comes to radiation exposure from multiple sources and that there is no safe level of man-made radiation. After we discuss how other people or populations on rare occasions have successfully faced such threats in the past, I'll begin to teach you how to maximize your healing response through regenerative healing techniques. By continually fortifying the internal cellular milieu in your body until your body induces The Regeneration Effect™,[337, 338, 339] you and your family will begin to push back against these constant low-level radiation exposures.

In *Fukushima Meltdown & Modern Radiation* "Part I, No Singing in the Black Rain," I began teaching you how you are being exposed to man-made radiation. In Part II, "Understanding How to Protect Your Family," you will learn how others have successfully dealt with the nature of nuclear threats. Finally in Part III, "Protecting Your Family," I will share very straightforward, individualized, easy to implement, cost effective, common sense daily programs you can undertake according to your family's budget.

In the aftermath of a nuclear accident, every ounce of prevention is vastly more precious than endless pounds of cure.

John W. Apsley

Chapter Three

Preventive Measures

In Chapter 1, I tell the story of two Nagasaki hospitals, each a little over a mile from ground zero when the atomic bomb was dropped. In this chapter, I will give you more detail about how the physician at the first hospital saved people's lives. And, I will use the learning from that experience to facilitate your understanding of how to protect yourself and your family.

In order of lethality, the first atomic bomb explosions in Nagasaki produced three deadly by-products as they converted uranium into pure energy: searing heat that for a split second rivaled that of the outer surface of the Sun, an extreme burst of gamma rays, and radioactive fallout.

The gamma rays produced vast quantities of radical oxygen species (ROS) in all surviving victims exposed to the blast. As ROS collides with tissues it will melt them, but when ROS collides with other ROS, they tend to cancel each other out. So for many present in the outskirts to ground zero, the huge production of ROS internally would have tended to cancel each other out even as it killed others closer in instantly. Those who survived likely did so in part according to the then unknown first principle of The Petkau Effect, which applies only to short bursts of intense radiation. Many of the survivors were expected to die rapidly within the following days and weeks.

As expected, rapid death was the overwhelming outcome to many of the staff and patients at the second hospital 180° across ground zero from St. Francis Hospital. Yet, St. Francis Hospital's novel diet therapy appeared able to completely protect all hospital staff members, as well as most patients.[340]

The second principle of The Petkau Effect is that the long-term exposure from the inhaled and ingested radioactive particles would have likely resulted in death over the following days, weeks, months and years. This, too, is what happened at the other hospital across the way. Yet, St. Francis Hospital's simple fare was apparently able to completely quench any lasting radiation sickness caused by radioactive particles.[341]

Our body's ability to cope with lethal radiation exposure is called our innate resistance. Each person's innate resistance depends on:

- ✓ The specific kind of radionuclide exposure and their respective yields of ROS and secondary pro-inflammatory agents.
- ✓ The quantity of radioactive body burden and their respective yields of ROS and secondary pro-inflammatory agents.
- ✓ The length of time present in our body.
- ✓ Antioxidant reserves in our body to antidote the ROS.
- ✓ The body's capacity to eliminate the radionuclides as quickly as possible and quench inflammation.
- ✓ Our ability to heal.

Therefore, the key objective in treating exposures to radiation and in preventing its onslaught upon human cells, tissues and organs, is to swiftly and comprehensively address all six criteria above. The clues to how this may be accomplished were first uncovered in the true-life historical experiences of an amazing group of 1945 Nagasaki Japanese survivors in the aftermath of the atomic bomb.

It is astounding that the simple fare utilized by St. Francis Hospital managed to successfully neutralize all three lethal forces in those who survived the initial moments of the carnage. We turn once again to the initial historical moments in the final hours of WWII where radio protection was first discovered in the medical setting:

> *In August 9th, 1945, the 2nd atomic bomb was dropped on Nagasaki. At the time, physician Tatuichirou Akizuki, worked with 20 employees, caring for 70 tuberculosis patients in Uragami Daiichi Hospital (St. Francis Hospital) located about 1.4km away from the hypocenter. However, these people, including Dr. Akizuki, escaped from death caused by acute radiation damage. Dr. Akizuki conjectured that the reason there was no nuclear bomb disease was that these people had consumed cups of wakame miso soup (Miso soup with garnish of wakame seaweed) every day.*[342]

Since then, many have also pointed out that the "Akizuki Diet" restricted all refined carbohydrates, candies and sweets. Rice was the main staple alongside fermented soy dishes.

The following is a detailed list of the lifesaving foods utilized at St. Francis Hospital:

- ✓ Miso, tofu, Tempeh and tamari (soy sauce)[343, 344, 345, 346, 347, 348, 349, 350]
- ✓ Rice[351, 352]

- ✓ Tea beverages[353, 354]
- ✓ Chinese cabbage[355, 356, 357, 358]
- ✓ Raw or lightly cooked sea vegetables[359, 360, 361, 362, 363, 364]
- ✓ Carrots and Hokkaido pumpkin[365]
- ✓ Pickles - low salt with living fermentative bacteria (probiotics)
- ✓ Mushrooms[366, 367]
- ✓ Green leafy vegetables when available[368]
- ✓ Contrary to some reports, it was likely that available fruits - high in antioxidants - were also consumed, such as raw Mikan, Kinkan, Nashi Ichigo and Ume.[369, 370]

Lessons Learned: Diet, Water and Air

The radiation burns, both externally and internally, were extreme in those who survived, yet the Akizuki Diet managed to save most. So, what was it about the simple diet that saved so many?

The survivors accomplished an amazing feat by implementing four practices:

- ✓ They undertook preventive measures to lessen ongoing radiation exposure
- ✓ They were administered select antidotes to the radiation
- ✓ They eliminated their body burden of radioactive particles via chelation agents

✓ They healed or regenerated their internal and external burned cells, tissues and organs

Perhaps the most significant preventative measure practiced by the Nagasaki survivors and staff members at St. Francis Hospital was their practice of eating low on the food chain. By eating a vegetarian diet with no animal products such as red meat and milk, their exposure to radioactive particles grew less and less as time wore on.

The top priority is to lessen your exposure as much as possible and avoid long-term contamination as much as possible. For example, eat low in the food chain focusing on nutrient rich foods. This means putting forth the effort to eat predominantly whole uncontaminated grains, beans, nuts, seeds, sea vegetables, vegetables and fruits.

One of the main staples of the past and present Japanese diet is rice, which resides at the bottom of the food chain. If St. Francis used fresh uncontaminated brown rice as opposed to polished white rice, the rice's content of phytates, B-Complex vitamins, at least one heat stable antioxidant enzyme, and select phenolics would also have aided in eliminating radionuclides from the body.[371, 372, 373]

Radionuclides bioaccumulate each time they are consumed in the food chain. For example, a cow eating contaminated grass and drinking contaminated water over its lifetime will bioaccumulate particles meaning that the meat from the cow, which is higher in the food chain than the grass the cow eats, will have higher concentrations of radionuclides than found in the grasses consumed.

Food Selections are Critical

Nutrient rich foods include those with high mineral content, such as uncontaminated sea vegetables. Therefore, taking appropriate amounts of select minerals to help thwart tissue absorption and deposition of radionuclides can also be extremely important and is discussed later in this book.[374]

Today, due to the large number of radionuclides that have contaminated the globe both pre-Fukushima and now post-Fukushima,[375] it is important to follow the below practices as much as possible:

As time passes, bioaccumulation will ebb and surge with escalating levels of the two most insidious radionuclides, 137Cs and 90Sr. These two have the greatest potential to contribute to our chronic degeneration. To combat their effect, whenever possible, eat low on the food chain and avoid meats, eggs and dairy products, with the exception of aged cheeses or dairy products imported from southern Italy or the southern hemisphere.[376, 377, 378, 379, 380] Alternatively, you may attempt to decontaminate milk, buttermilk, yogurt, sour cream, ice cream or eggs using one of the following techniques:

- ✓ Mix ¼ teaspoon of edible clay per cup of dairy or per egg (leaves no "flavor after taste")
- ✓ Mix or blend 100mg calcium alginate per cup of dairy or per egg
- ✓ Mix 100mg pectin per cup of dairy or per egg

Avoid Pacific seafood caught above the equator. As of early June 2011, the amount of oceanic contamination coming out of Fukushima already exceeds 10 times that of the entire Chernobyl Catastrophe, with an end nowhere in sight.[381, 382, 383,

[384] For example, a recent report covering the months of June through July 2011 by the Chinese State Oceanic Administration revealed that there were multiple oceanic hot spots for 137Cs and 90Sr up to 500 miles off the coast of Fukushima. The report went on to state that the levels of 90Sr were up to 10 times higher than coastal Chinese waters, but astonishingly up to 300 times higher for 137Cs compared to coastal Chinese waters.[385] Seafood caught in the eastern northern Pacific may be safe for several months after the March 2011 event, but it is now clear that vast regions have been exposed to fallout making it difficult to avoid all risk. Instead, buy North Atlantic seafood.[386]

Wash all fresh produce the moment you arrive home from the grocery store. Wash (soak) the outer layer of fresh produce in a sink filled with water and baking soda. Simply fill a sink half way with filtered tap water and add in three tablespoons of baking soda. You can also pull radionuclides off of foods by putting ¼ cup magnetic clay into the sink full of water. Soak in either solution for ten minutes.

Taking a broad-spectrum multi-mineral supplement with each meal might be wise in addition to specific minerals which target the most important threats of radionuclides.

Consume North Atlantic-sourced kelp tablets daily. They are high in iodine, potassium, calcium and chlorophyll which can prevent the uptake of 131-I and other radionuclides.

Water Filtration is Critical

In contrast to Japan, only above ground water reservoirs are in danger of becoming contaminated with radioactive particles here in North America.[387] The water table (i.e., well water) would not be threatened because most radionuclides adhere for long time periods upon the first few centimeters of soils, especially if rich in clay.

Drinking Water - In late June of 2011, a debate was raging between the Environmental Protection Agency (EPA) and the Nuclear Regulatory Commission (NRC). It concerned the dramatic rise in radioactivity across the United States public drinking water system. Up until the Fukushima Catastrophe, the upward allowable dose in the public water supplies was 4 millirems per year. Now that the United States has received significant fallout from Fukushima Catastrophe, the EPA is unable to protect the United States public water supply other than to simply raise the permissible limits of radiation to 500 millirems per year![388] What part of the scientifically established fact that, "There is no known safe level of radiation" does the EPA not understand? If your tap water source is not well water, consider a multi-stage water filtration system that incorporates both charcoal and reverse osmosis (RO).

For showers, use a Vitamin C or Zeolite based shower head filter. For baths, use ½ teaspoon of inexpensive ascorbic acid per bath tub, or 1 cup of magnetic clay.

Air Filtration is Critical

If your home is located near nuclear power plants, on the west coast of the United States or in other areas receiving significant levels of airborne radiation, consider HEPA filtration systems. If your car is equipped with an air conditioner, have the air filter switched out on a frequent basis.

Mineral Supplements May Block Entry of Radionuclides

You can prevent radionuclides from absorbing into the depths of the body by taking select mineral supplements.

Iodine for Thyroid Protection

When the fuel rods in a nuclear power plant accident begin to meltdown, large releases of radioactive iodine are spewed into the air. The meltdown can sometimes slow and then resume, and then slow again until all the fuel has melted. In such cases, 131-I can continue to be released in waves until all the fuel has melted. Halogens (such as iodine) like to turn into gases, just like chlorine prefers the gaseous state. 131-I is very dangerous when released during meltdowns, because once it becomes airborne, it can travel great distances, even across the globe.

During the times that 131-I is released, it will easily come back down to earth during rainstorms. For the next 80 days or so, in regions doused with 131-I, it becomes vital to attempt to prevent radioactive iodine from becoming absorbed into our tissues. Staying out of the rain is the first order of business. Taking a prudent dose of good iodine is the second order of business.[389]

One of the best ways to do this is to super saturate the body with natural iodine from North Atlantic Kelp, if there is no allergy or sensitivity to taking natural iodine supplements. Once the body is saturated with the natural iodine, the body turns off systems that transport any more iodine into the body. Also, once the body is saturated with natural iodine, it typically turns up the systems that export iodine out of the body. Taking natural iodine supplements is a prudent measure to ward off 131-I contamination if administered properly.[390]

There are many forms of iodine supplements discussed below, and there are added benefits to taking sea vegetables which are high in iodine, such as kelp.

Besides protecting us from 131-I, kelp may help protect us from at least two other radioactive elements of great import frequently released during a nuclear power plant accident. More specifically, edible seaweeds are excellent chelators (removers) of toxic radioactive cesium (137Cs and 134Cs) and radioactive strontium (90Sr and 89Sr) from the body, especially if you consume a high fiber diet (i.e., pectin from fruits).[391, 392, 393]

Below is an excerpt from a study completed by Yamamoto:

> *We conducted an animal experiment to determine how dietary seaweeds rich in iodine and dietary fibers suppress radioactive iodine uptake by the thyroid, using mice and four kinds of experimental diets, three with 1% or 2% powdered fronds of the kelp Laminaria religiosa and 2% powdered laver Porphyra yezoensis, and one with cellulose. Iodine content of a hot-water extract of the kelp was 0.530 +/- 0.001%, and its dietary fiber (DF) values were 52.8 +/- 1.2%. Iodine in an extract of the laver was 0.008 +/- 0.001%, and its DF values were 41.4% +/- 0.7%. A statistically significant reduction of 125I uptake by the thyroid, 3 hours after intragastric administration of the radionuclide at a dosage of 18.5 kBq or 185 kBq in 0.3 ml aqueous solution per mouse, was observed in mice previously fed the experimental diets containing 1% and 2% kelp during periods varying from 24 hours to 7 days. The degree of the suppression was observed to depend on the amount of iodine in the diet or in the injected sample, no matter whether organic or inorganic, judging from the results of an additional experiment.*

> *Thus, we conclude that previously fed iodine-rich material, especially dietary seaweeds rich in iodine and other minerals, vitamins, and beta-carotene, such as kelps or laver supplemented with inorganic iodine, may be effective in prevention of internal radiation injury of the thyroid.*[394]

Sea vegetables high in iodine have been used for centuries by millions of folks as a part of their regular diet. Iodine is an essential element, so we must consume proper amounts daily. For example, there are a few organs in the body that require a lot of iodine daily - the thyroid gland, gonads and breast tissues.[395] Some of the most healthy folks in the world consume approximately 13,000mcg (13mg) daily of iodine.[396] That is almost *one hundred times* the "recommended" daily dosage and over ten times the "upward" dosage range suggested by United States government authorities.[397]

For an average size woman, daily requirements for the thyroid gland amount to 50mcg iodine alone. But what may be surprising to many is the much higher amounts needed by a woman's breast tissues and ovaries, which collectively require up to 3,000mcg (3mg) daily. For men, there is solid evidence intake should be at least 1,000mcg (1mg) daily, unless they are sensitive to the mineral.[398]

So, despite misinformation to the contrary, if one has no known allergy to shellfish or iodide, rational supplementation with food-based iodine is a good thing.[399, 400]

Iodine supplementation can be a little tricky. In a nuclear accident crisis, your doctor may wish to have you take large doses of iodine for a short period of time. In situations where there is sufficient time, it is more prudent to take lower dosages of iodine, and work up to the larger daily dosages as tolerance permits. Many adults do best by only taking 200mcg daily to start, and then work up in 200mcg increments to the optimal level as instructed by their physician.[401]

Under normal circumstances, physicians typically run a simple iodine loading test to help determine if a patient needs to take iodine. In iodine deficiency, the body will be on the lookout for any source of iodine it comes into contact with. Anyone can perform a simple test with a liquid iodine such as Lugo's solution (potassium iodide). The forearm is used where no hair is growing. Next, liquid iodine solution is "painted" over a two-inch square patch on the forearm. The skin will quickly turn yellow from the iodine. If the body is deficient in iodine, the yellow will disappear within 24 hours.

Experienced holistic physicians knowledgeable in "iodine loading therapy" often start their adult patients with one kelp tablet per day for three days to determine patient tolerance. If tolerance to one tablet of kelp daily is determined, then the dosage after three days is raised by the physician to one tablet per meal (3 per day). If tolerance remains intact, after three more days two (2) tablets per meal are often suggested. If tolerance remains intact after three days, three (3) tablets per meal are recommended. In this manner, most adult patients easily achieve taking five (5) tablets or more of kelp per meal in about one month.

Holistic physicians may use up to ten times or more of the female dose to treat chronic fatigue and advanced Fibromyalgia with great success (50mg to 100mg per day).[402] Also, holistic physicians understand the value of detoxifying their patients on a regular basis. Some of the more common toxic elements we consume in our white bread products and in our tap water are bromide, chloride and fluoride. These three often interfere with normal thyroid function, and/or get stored away in vital and non-vital tissues.[403] Taking optimal amounts of natural iodine helps the body detoxify these toxic halides out of the body.[404] But beware - these toxic halides may exit through the skin, confusing folks that they are experiencing a mild allergic reaction to the iodine. To the contrary, this release of toxic elements will soon pass, especially if the individual is bathing frequently, taking vitamin C and keeping well hydrated.

Be aware of potential iodine sensitivity. When high levels of iodine are taken too abruptly, toxins may exit "en masse" so quickly that temporary skin rashes, minor hair loss, congestion, scratchy throat, or very rarely, even asthmatic reactions may arise.

Holistic physicians will neutralize this sensitivity with up to 3,000mg daily of Vitamin C (1,000mg in three divided doses, such as 1,000mg with each meal).[405] But by simply discontinuing the iodine supplement for several days, skin or hair issues should quickly clear up on their own. Anyone experiencing anything more dramatic should check in with their doctor right away.

In review, by increasing iodine intake *slowly* and according to *tolerance,* most folks may protect themselves from radioactive iodine.

For people with sensitivity to iodine, if symptoms clear after discontinuing iodine intake, this suggests that there may be a way to slowly add sea vegetables back into ones diet. Again, Vitamin C may be the key.

Under a doctor's supervision, taking ¼ of a tablet of kelp daily may be well tolerated in those who have experienced iodine sensitivity in the past. By remaining on 3,000mg of Vitamin C daily, every three days it may be possible to increase iodine intake by another ¼ kelp tablet daily. In this manner, many previously iodine-sensitive folks will slowly work up to one (1) tablet daily. Over time, most folks can up their dosage to the full amount suggested above, although these folks must proceed much more slowly than other people. Staying on 3,000mg of Vitamin C per day is often the key to success. Several months down the road, one initially sensitive to iodine may find themselves able to take 400mcg to 1,000mcg daily if they use patience. In the rare event that any intake of iodide causes resumption of symptoms, including minor hair loss, this may help your doctor identify an underlying thyroid disorder.

There are several kinds of thyroid disorders doctors may successfully treat by natural means. These thyroid disorders are beyond the scope of this book, but should be addressed if present.

Potassium and Calcium Supplements

Potassium may be taken (99mg per meal) to help thwart 137Cs absorption.[406, 407] Also, taking calcium supplements in the form of uncontaminated, high grade bone meal from the southern hemisphere can help prevent the absorption of 90Sr.[408, 409] One such high quality bone meal product is Calcium Hydroxy-apatite. This high-end product will help protect against bone penetration of both 90Sr as well as radioactive uranium (234/238U). Three (3) per meal (or as labeled) is the suggested dose for adults. Young adults and older children may take two (2) per meal, and one (1) per meal for the very young in juice or other liquid may be appropriate.[410] Specifically, the International Commission for Radiological Protection (ICRP) conducted a study that confirmed those not ingesting adequate levels of minerals such as calcium were more vulnerable to absorbing and retaining higher levels of radionuclides:

> *Within the framework of a Coordinated Research Project (CRP) organized by the International Atomic Energy Agency,*

Vienna, the daily dietary intakes of seven elements by adult populations living in nine Asian countries were estimated. The countries that participated in the study were Bangladesh, China, India, Indonesia, Japan, Pakistan, Philippines, South Korea (Republic of Korea, ROK), and Vietnam and together they represented more than half of the world population. The seven elements studied were calcium, cesium, iodine, potassium, strontium, thorium, and uranium. These elements have chemical and biological similarity to some of the radionuclides abundantly encountered during nuclear power production and therefore data on these elements could provide important information on their biokinetic behavior... The median daily dietary intakes for the adult Asian population were found to be 0.45 g calcium, 7 microg cesium, 90 microg iodine, 1.75 g potassium, 1.65 mg strontium, 1 microg thorium, and 1 microg uranium. When compared with the intakes proposed for ICRP Reference Man by International Commission for Radiological Protection, these intakes were lower by factors of 0.41 for calcium, 0.7 for cesium, 0.45 for iodine, 0.53 for potassium, 0.87 for strontium, 0.33 for thorium, and 0.52 for uranium. The lower daily intakes of calcium, cesium, and iodine by the Asian population could be due to significantly lower consumption of milk and milk products, which are rich in these elements. The significantly lower intake of calcium in most of the Asian countries may lead to higher uptake of fission nuclide 90Sr and could result in perhaps higher internal radiation dose...[411]

Selenium, Zinc, Copper and Manganese Supplements

Lastly, selenium, zinc, copper and manganese are extremely critical minerals since they activate four of the most important antioxidant enzyme systems of the body responsible for neutralizing radiation exposure - Glutathione peroxidase (GPx), methionine reductase, thioredoxin and superoxide dismutase (S.O.D.). Coincidently, Vitamin C also stimulates production of most of these antioxidant systems as well.[412,413] Prioritizing the restoration and optimization of antioxidant enzymes over non-enzyme antioxidants has greater value to the host because the former works many orders of magnitude faster at neutralizing ROS than non-enzyme antioxidants.[414]

Let food be thy medicine and medicine be thy food.

Hippocrates

Chapter Four

Antioxidants and Other Hot Particle Quenchers

The Akizuki Diet was rich in antioxidants. As we know from the last chapter, antioxidants neutralize much of the ionizing destruction emitted by radionuclides once they enter the body. The key is to take supplements to step-up the antioxidant systems plus the more powerful and ubiquitous non-enzymatic antioxidants.

Perhaps the most powerful non-enzymatic radio-protective antioxidants are select omega 3 oils. Rice-koji-miso, likely a frequent member of the Akizuki Diet, is rich in omega 3 ethyl esters.[415] Omega 3 oils also quench inflammation.

Vitamin C is a key nutrient that activates key enzymatic antioxidant systems of the body.[416] Enzymatic antioxidant systems operate billions of times faster than non-enzymatic antioxidants at normal body temperatures.[417] Plus, the use of lightly cooked cabbage and mustard family vegetables, green tea, and grape wines or fresh grapes would have offered heat-stable isothiocyanates, EGCG (active ingredient in green tea) and resveratrol that all step-up key enzymatic antioxidant systems via Nrf2, which is covered more extensively later in this chapter.[418, 419, 420]

Lastly, fermented microbes likely aid both neutralization of the radiation as well as provide enhancement to the patient's immune system. Properly prepared Miso soup (fermented soy) with added sea vegetables and root vegetables (often pickled), and mushrooms, brown rice and tea beverages offer an anti-radiation power-meal of highly potent antioxidants.[421]

Ionizing radiation produces vast amounts of radical oxygen species (ROS) which must be checked. The key ROS culprits are super oxide radical (O^-), hydroxyl radical (OH^-), and hydrogen peroxide (H_2O_2). Over the next century, hundreds of millions if not billions of folks will inhale or ingest radio-nuclides from the Fukushima fallout causing damage to their cells, tissues and organs when they produce ROS. Fortunately, we have a highly evolved but rate limited[422] antioxidant system within our bodies to antidote ROS. This system is an interconnected system composed of both proteins (i.e., enzymes) as well as select nutrients. Basically, there are four conditions that optimize antioxidant function in our bodies:

- ✓ The antioxidant enzymes must all work together to keep up with the lethal effects of radiation poisoning.[423]
- ✓ The antioxidant enzymes systems must also work together with select nutrients to keep up with lethal effects of radiation poisoning.[424, 425] For example, the co-enzymated B-Complex vitamins and reduced CoQ10 (i.e., CoQ10(H) or Ubiquinol), are essential to many antioxidant enzymes systems such as Methionine reductase and endothelial S.O.D. respectively.[426, 427]
- ✓ Antioxidant nutrients must work together with other antioxidant nutrients to stay fully charged and get recharged, when facing the lethal effects from radiation poisoning.[428, 429] For example, selenium is ambogenic[430] with Vitamin E, "spent"[431] Vitamin E is recharged by Vitamin C and/or CoQ10(H) at cell membranes,[432, 433]

"spent" Vitamin C is recharged by Lipoic Acid and glutathione,[434, 435] and antioxidant enzymes are optimally activated up to 20 times by heat and/or "Vitagenes" of which the amino acid Acetyl-L-Carnitine (ALCAR) is a key initiator.[436, 437]

✓ At the cell and below the cell level, antioxidants must be matched according to their residence within the cells. Some antioxidants play greater or lesser roles in the cell membranes, the cell mitochondria (the engines of our metabolism), or the cell nucleus (which houses our genetic core).

All four of the above must work together to help us cope with radiation fallout from Fukushima. Also, select herbal remedies can aid in quickly establishing optimal levels of antioxidant enzyme systems, as indicated below.

As mentioned above, enzymes work billions of times faster than nutrients at normal body temperature. So, it is best to first concentrate efforts to keep our antioxidant enzymes happy, content and well stocked. ROS are the primary villain for both the Petkau Effect as well as for genetic defects. Radionuclides ionize our tissues and produce lethal quantities of ROS sooner or later. It is now known that nuclear plant accidents will deplete reserves of antidotes (antioxidants) that neutralize ROS in those exposed.[438] Therefore, if you have been exposed to radiation, it is critical to keep the antioxidant reserves at maximum levels.[439]

There are five very important antioxidant enzymes systems within our cells. These antioxidant systems quench the most lethal ROS produced by ionizing radiation, namely super oxide radical (O^-), hydroxyl radical (OH^-) and hydrogen peroxide (H_2O_2). Superoxide Dismutase or S.O.D., Catalase, the Glutathione family of antioxidant enzymes, the Methionine Reductase group of antioxidant enzymes, plus

Thioredoxin achieve this. The key genes involved to their respective optimal production and cellular reserves are collectively known as Nrf2.[440] The importance of Nrf2 in defeating radiation poisoning cannot be overstated, and my book will drive this point home with practical solutions for how to optimize your Nrf2 function. A critical function of these enzymes systems is to repair DNA damage (both SSB and DSB), but optimal oxygen saturation into the cells appears to be required.[441, 442, 443] So taking daily long walks in unpolluted fresh air is a good idea.

The following descriptions respectively provide more highlights to these five critical high rate radiation antidote systems:

S.O.D. is a group of three slightly different enzymes that together comprise the fifth most common protein that exists within our bodies. S.O.D. plays a huge role in every cell of our body by quenching arguably the most lethal oxygen radical - namely super oxide radical (O^-). Each kind of S.O.D. enzyme is different from its other forms by the required mineral it must have to fully operate as an antioxidant. There is Zinc dependent, Copper dependent, and Manganese dependent S.O.D. Fortunately, S.O.D. typically increases in numbers when there are plenty of minerals, select vegetables, Vitamin C, certain herbs[444] and precise amino acids available from the diet. Also, CoQ10(H) may compensate for deficits in S.O.D. functions.[445]

Catalase is the next antioxidant enzyme of great importance. It will also automatically increase its numbers in a rapid manner when needed. If you ingest enough essential amino acids from sources such as whey products (rich in cystine and cysteine) or food grade algae products (rich in minerals such as zinc) and other Nrf2 activating factors, both S.O.D. and catalase enzymes groups should be able to keep up with emergencies such as being exposed to nuclear fallout particles.[446, 447]

Glutathione is a tripeptide, meaning it is composed of three amino acids. There are five families of antioxidant enzymes in our bodies that require glutathione and all act to quench hydrogen peroxide (H_2O_2). These five antioxidant enzyme systems can be sluggish in catching up in an emergency. Yet, these enzymes are absolutely essential to keep us ahead of the lethal effects of radiation poisoning plus all other chemical insults coming our way. Therefore, building up reserves of glutathione takes first priority over the two above groups (S.O.D. and Catalase), since the latter two appear to have less difficulty keeping up.[448, 449] NAC, glycine and glutamine are required amino acids to form glutathione, but melatonin is the key determinant to produce glutathione internally within cells. Also, CoQ10(H) may compensate for deficits in Glutathione functions.[450]

Methionine (synthase) Reductase is essential for quenching hydroxyl radical (OH^-). Both Glutathione peroxidase (GPx) and Methionine reductase require selenium, so selenium methionate is an excellent supporting nutraceutical to both enzymes families. Other important optimizers which help reactivate spent methionine reductase are methionine, folic acid and Vitamin B-12.[451]

Thioredoxin is a major player in redox recycling pools, and therefore regenerates antioxidant systems. It is a master regulator to prevent heart ROS injury, a central cause of Chernobyl Heart or cardiac hypertrophy.[452] Specifically, it teams with glutathione to defeat ROS, and is also essential for optimal protection to our genetic and neural integrity.[453] Thioredoxin levels in the body are optimized by ingesting members of the cabbage family including wasabi, as well as by curcumin.[454, 455, 456, 457]

Antidoting the Petkau Effect

Starting with Cell Membrane (Lipid) Protection, we now turn to neutralizing the Petkau Effect. The top gun to quench ROS among the five antioxidant enzymes systems discussed above appears to be the Thioredoxin group (which is fat soluble), in close alliance with the glutathione family. In order of strength for the non-enzymatic antioxidants, krill oil reigns supreme for lowering the risks from the Petkau Effect. It is the best form of the omega 3 oils currently available. Krill oil is 48 times more powerful than omega 3 from fish oils and 34 times more powerful than CoQ10 on the ORAC scale.[458, 459, 460, 461] Besides being more easily digested than fish oils, it is also rich in *natural* astaxanthin (as opposed to synthetic astaxanthin derived from petrochemicals), the most powerful fat soluble carotenoid discovered to date. It is 550 times more powerful than Vitamin E alone.[462] Make sure your krill oil is sourced from the uncontaminated Antarctic Ocean.

The next most important nutrient to neutralize the Petkau Effect would be CoQ10(H),[463, 464] then R-alpha lipoic acid (R-ALA),[465] next liposomal (i.e., fat-soluble) Vitamin C, selenium,[466, 467] and finally all natural, full spectrum, Vitamin E.[468, 469, 470]

Antidoting the Genetic Damage via HRR & NHEJ

Cell Nucleus Protection addresses the genetic damage from radiation. This threat is deflected by many of the above antioxidant enzyme systems, plus the perennial N-Acetyl-Cysteine (NAC) + Selenium (Se) + melatonin combination.[471]

Antioxidant Enzyme Systems are key to protecting the vital roles of two key DNA repair enzymes, abbreviated HRR and NHEJ. This is because both HRR and NHEJ are highly vulnerable to ROS.[472] By preventing and quickly quenching ROS within the genetic core, the integrity of HRR and NHEJ are assured enabling optimal DNA repair to go efficiently forward.[473]

Melatonin is the premier antidote without equal for radiation poisoning.[474, 475, 476] First, melatonin stimulates the production of the SOD family of antioxidant enzymes, catalase *and* the glutathione family of enzymes, by way of bolstering Nrf2.[477, 478] Second, melatonin is essential for restoring and building up cellular reserves of glutathione, the central molecule to all glutathione antioxidant enzyme family members.[479, 480] Melatonin is also essential to "prime start" repair to the genetic core once radiation poisoning has occurred, including damage done to our delicate nervous system, a favorite target of radioactive particles.[481, 482, 483] Finally, melatonin single-handedly and directly quenches nearly all forms of ROS, including singlet oxygen (O^-), hydroxyl radical (OH^-), hydrogen peroxide (H_2O_2), nitric oxide (NO), peroxynitrous acid, and the most pro-inflammatory of all - peroxynitrite anion (ONOO-).

This is one highly cost-effective radioprotective supplement wise people should take just before bedtime.

After melatonin, NAC is perhaps the most versatile and powerful quencher of ionizing radiation because it does work on both the fat as well as the genetic defenses. For example, NAC offers superior protection from toxic metals (which often disturb genetic functions)[484] and other poisons.[485, 486]

NAC may be used indefinitely as long as no sensitivity arises (i.e., light skin rashes). In this manner, NAC may be used daily as it is a harmless amino acid our bodies will use to establish and maintain antioxidant defenses. For folks who discover they are sensitive to NAC, substitute with high-quality Whey products (free from radioactive particles).[487, 488]

Organic Selenium as selenomethionate, selenocysteine or in other organic forms (such as when grown into kelp or other foods) is an exceptional quencher of radiation toxicity.[489] It works with NAC and melatonin to create the glutathione and thioredoxin family of enzymes. Both are critical anti-oxidant enzyme systems each cell uses to successfully defend against radiation.[490, 491, 492, 493, 494, 495]

Preventing Ionizing Radiation from Inducing Chronic Degenerative Diseases

Cell Mitochondria Protection addresses the main energy production center of the body. All chronic degenerative diseases known to this author involve various levels of compromise to the vital mitochondria.[496] Two sets of antioxidants are intimately involved with protecting the vital mitochondria: (a) antioxidant enzymes and (b) non-enzymatic antioxidants.

As previously discussed, top priority must be given to five antioxidant enzyme systems in the body:

1. The S.O.D. system of three specific enzymes: Zinc-S.O.D. (ZnS.O.D.), Copper-S.O.D. (CuS.O.D.) and Manganese-S.O.D. (MnS.O.D.). To maximize the antioxidant power of S.O.D., zinc, copper and manganese must be supplied in the diet or specifically supplemented.[497] Collectively, S.O.D. forms the fifth most common protein in the body enabling broad-spectrum mitochondrial protection.

2. Catalase.

3. The glutathione system of enzymes.

4. Methionine reductase.

5. The Thioredoxin family of enzymes.

As mentioned above, Nrf2 is the key to optimal production of S.O.D., catalase and both the glutathione and thioredoxin antioxidant systems in the body. To maximize its powers, cruciferous vegetables such as cabbage and green tea significantly enhance Nrf2 levels and function, as do the herbal extracts curcumin and resveratrol.[498, 499, 500, 501] It appears that adequate levels of thyroid hormone may also play a significant role in Nrf2 production and function.[502]

Critical non-enzymatic antioxidants of highest importance for protecting the mitochondria are the omega 3 oils, CoQ10(H), lipoic acid and natural Vitamin E.

The primary cause of disease is corruption of the harmony of mineral elements in the Biosphere. If traces of perennial radionuclides pervade our air and cover our soils, food and water will sooner or later become equally corrupt. Could anything else better define the verse - Earth to earth, ashes to ashes, dust to dust?

John W. Apsley

Chapter Five

Radiation Elimination

Many people will unknowingly find themselves eating radioactively contaminated foods on a regular basis. Current Environmental Protection Agency (EPA) limits on permissible levels of radionuclides in our foods is shameful, but a fact of our modern, nuclear age. For example, if radiation is allowed in our drinking water, it will be ever present in foods grown using the water.

The EPA currently publishes permissible levels of radiation in rain water at less than 3 pCi/L. Once in the food chain, or where crops grow, cattle are raised, or dairy herds are kept, it will remain in the food chain for decades. Keep in mind that children are three to 10 times or more susceptible to ingesting radiation poisons than adults.

On March 22nd, Richmond, CA received astounding radiation levels of 138 pCi/L, and Boise, ID recorded the highest in the nation at 242 pCi/L. Levels of NW rain water also became astoundingly high throughout the month of March. Olympia, WA received rains with 41 times over the EPA permissible standards. On March 24th, Iodine-131 rose to 125 pCi/L. On March 25th, Portland, OR received 86.8 pCi/L. But on March 27th, Boise broke the record again with readings of 390 pCi/L, which is 130 times over permissible levels.[503]

In most cases, radioactive particles are radioactive metals that may be removed from the body (scientifically termed decorporation) by a process known as "chelation." In the aftermath of the atomic bomb dropped on Nagasaki and the Chernobyl Catastrophes, the Akizuki Diet again offers us considerable insight into how to eliminate (decorporate through chelation) the radionuclides (i.e., ***chelation*** - from the Greek which means a process using non-toxic carrier substances that "grab onto or claw into" toxic substances facilitating their elimination from the body). The Akizuki Diet provided chelating agents from non-polished rice (phytates), sea vegetables (alginate), fruits (pectin), cruciferous vegetables (sulfur containing reducing agents), and Miso (phytates, zybicolin or dipicolinic acid, which is closely related to picolinate).[504,505] In the aftermath of the Chernobyl Catastrophe, high-grade edible clays were also used with significant success.

You can choose among three separate strategies for chelating agents as described below.

1. The first is to prevent new radionuclides from entering into the human body by chelating to the particles as they travel down the intestinal track after ingestion.

2. The second is to remove radionuclides already present in the tissues from prior exposure. As mentioned above, the latter strategy is called decorporation.

3. The third strategy is to accomplish both of the above simultaneously as appropriate.

Diet → Bowel Elimination

There are several excellent all-natural tools for removing radioactive metals from foods as they are being digested. If taken with meals, high-grade edible clays, pectin and high fiber diets will help keep radionuclides from entering our bodies. If there is a source for uncontaminated sea vegetables and fresh water chlorella, their respective alginate and other chelation agents offer superior means to eliminate incoming radionuclides. The sections below describe these tools.

Cabbage Family Vegetables

By simply adding cabbage family members to your diet regularly, it appears possible to help prevent radionuclides unknowingly present in our foods from entering into the internal body.

For example, emerging evidence suggests that Chinese cabbage and other members of the cabbage family containing isothiocyanates will effectively bind to radionuclides such as 137Cs, 90Sr and cobalt (60Co) when they come into direct contact.[506, 507, 508]

Edible Clays

Calcium Bentonite

One of the more widely used food grade clays is Calcium Bentonite. It has the advantage of supplying extra calcium when removing other metals from the body. Other forms of edible clays may also chelate out essential calcium from the ingested foods. Even though the drug Prussian Blue may be more effective than bentonite in removing 137Cs, there are other advantages in favor of bentonite. First, it is just as non-toxic as Prussian Blue. Secondly, calcium bentonite offers calcium to the body, which would help lessen the G.I. absorption of 90Sr. Third, bentonite likely chelates many more types of radionuclides than Prussian Blue, due to its broad ion exchange spectrum. Fourth, it is available over-the-counter. And fifth, it is very economical.

> *Two experiments were performed with lactating dairy cattle to assess the efficacy of clay minerals and Prussian Blue (AFCF form) in controlling the transfer of dietary radiocaesium to milk. In Experiment 1, bentonite was included in the diet at 0, 300, 600 and 900 g d-1 and the transfer of radiocaesium from silage to milk was determined. Bentonite inclusion significantly (P less than 0.001) depressed the transfer of radiocaesium to milk with no benefit in increasing the dietary inclusion above 600 g d-1 when a 73% reduction was observed. In Experiment 2, the effectiveness of bentonite (300 g d-1), clinoptilolite (300 g d-1) and Prussian Blue (3 g d-1) as dietary additives was compared. All treatments significantly (P less than 0.001) depressed the transfer of dietary radiocaesium to milk. Clinoptilolite was less effective than bentonite and both treatments were considerably less effective than Prussian Blue, the reductions being 35%, 62% and 85% respectively.*[509]

Also, it is sometimes highly desirable to use the skin as a channel of elimination. The skin is our largest organ of the body. It is also an extremely important respiratory organ for our tissues closest to the surface. Toxins are typically eliminated through the skin. When the skin layers become overloaded with these toxins, not only does our skin fail to bring in optimal levels of oxygen into these tissues, but our entire elimination system begins to back-up. Therefore, it is important to keep our skin pores well cleaned.

One of the best ways to keep our skin healthy and the surrounding tissues well oxygenated, is to simply take a 30 minute hot bath several times a week with magnetic clay. If you do not have a home-wide water filter, use ¼ teaspoon of pure, cheap, vitamin C (ascorbic acid) per bath tub first. This eliminates the chlorine and fluorine residues. Then the magnetic clay can go to work to bind to toxic metals being excreted as you sweat. Just make sure you keep the water temperature as hot as possible, but enjoyable and never burning.

Altogether, edible and magnetic clays are superior removers of 137Cs. For example, calcium bentonite alone is known to remove up to 62% of the 137Cs present in the body of children.[510, 511]

Pectin

Another well used chelation agent of Chernobyl vintage is pectin from fruits. The scientific literature has utilized pectin in human children studies to determine how effective it is in cases where the radionuclides are already present in the child, as opposed to simply helping to prevent new entries of the radionuclides from the food supplies.

> *As a complement of standard radioprotective measures, apple-pectin preparations are given, especially in the Ukraine, to reduce the 137Cs uptake in the organism of children. The question has been raised: is oral pectin also useful when children receive radiologically clean food, or does this polysaccharide only act in binding 137Cs in the gut, blocking its intestinal absorption?*
>
> *In this case, pectin would be useless if radiologically clean food could be given. The study was a randomised, double blind placebo-controlled trial comparing the efficacy of a dry and*

milled apple-extract containing 15–16% pectin with a similar placebo-powder, in 64 children originating from the same group of contaminated villages of the Gomel oblast. The average 137Cs load was of about 30 Bq/kg bodyweight (BW). The trial was conducted during the simultaneous one-month stay in the sanatorium Silver Spring. In this clean radiological environment only radiologically "clean" food is given to the children.

The average reduction of the 137Cs levels in children receiving oral pectin powder was 62.6%, the reduction with "clean" food and placebo was 13.9%, the difference being statistically significant (p <0.01). The reduction of the 137Cs load is medically relevant, as no child in the placebo group reached values below 20 Bq/kg BW (which is considered by Bandazhevsky as potentially associated with specific pathological tissue damages), with an average value of 25.8 ± 0.8 Bq/kg. The highest value in the apple-pectin group was 15.4 Bq/kg, the average value being 11.3 ± 0.6 Bq/kg BW.[512]

In an nutshell, pectin is an excellent remover of 137Cs, one of the worst offending radionuclides we receive from fallout.[513, 514]

Probiotics

Acidophilus, Bifidus and other beneficial gut microbes, are excellent eliminators of radionuclides. Including these into the daily diet is simply an excellent idea, so long as the dairy sources used to grow and concentrate the microbes are from uncontaminated sources.[515, 516]

Alginate

Let's first take a look at the sea vegetable extract known as alginate, a polysaccharide or chain of sugar molecules similar to cellulose or starch. Alginate is an excellent remover of 90Sr.[517, 518, 519]

The Akizuki Diet made liberal use of Miso soup, which was typically loaded with sea vegetables. Miso is made through fermentation with soy beans. The fermentation process involves benign probiotics that produce enzymes to help break down the soybean into the delicious products we know as Miso, soy sauce and other fermented soy products. It turns out that enzymes these probiotics make appear to have a very positive secondary effect on the sea vegetables when placed into the Miso soup. For example, sea vegetables are rich in alginate and are already well known to chelate to food borne radionuclides in both animal and human studies. Alginates reduce the absorption of 90Sr by up to 78%. So the next question is, can this level of reduced absorption be improved upon?

It is conceivable that sea vegetables rich in alginate may undergo enzymatic hydrolysis during the cooking process to break down the alginate into an array of smaller chelating fragments.[520, 521, 522] If true, the increased surface area of these chelating fragments should further reduce G.I. 90Sr absorption above that of whole alginate. Indeed, it appears that such biologically active chelating fragments may offer an extra 1% to 31% increase in absorption efficacy.[523]

Two required factors would remain for positive effects. First, the Miso soup containing the sea vegetables should be thoroughly chewed to glean the most from the sea vegetable components. Second, do not use prolonged high heat to cook the Miso soup/sea vegetable mix. High heat would destroy the enzymes. As a result, it is necessary to properly prepare Miso soup as previously described.

Sea vegetables form a huge industry for Japan. As previously discussed, collected sea vegetables in and around the greater Japanese oceanic waters are now unsuitable for human consumption. Sea weeds collected as foodstuffs around the east coast of China and Korea are likely to also become unsuitable for human consumption. Sea vegetables grown in uncontaminated water elsewhere will remain superior chelation tools for removing radioactive poisons from our bodies.

Chlorella

Chlorella has a unique cell wall, that when cracked via special processes, provides an excellence surface area to bind to radionuclides. For example, chlorella is a superior eliminator of radioactive uranium (239U).[524] Chlorella is chiefly grown in Taiwan as well as Japan. So these sources of chlorella are no longer suitable for human consumption.

Blood ➔ Urine Elimination

High Grade Zeolite (super activated clinoptilolite)

On special occasions where body radioactive particle burdens may be quite high, daily use (for one month) of super activated Zeolite may be prudent. Thereafter, using less expensive calcium bentonite as follow-up would lessen the chance of future calcium malabsorption, while maintaining progress.

> *Effective treatment of chronic illness resulting from the long-term buildup of heavy metals in the body, such as chelation therapy, presents numerous clinical challenges, including undesirable side effects and unpredictable efficacy. Use of a*

naturally occurring zeolite, clinoptilolite, to remove these toxic substances may offer an efficacious and safe alternative to the traditional approaches. This study was designed to evaluate the ability of activated clinoptilolite suspended in water (ACS) to remove heavy metals from the body through urinary excretion without the undesirable removal of physiologically important electrolytes. The protocol utilized two treatment groups, each consisting of eleven healthy men aged 36 to 70 years. Volunteers were given a commercially available version of the study substance for seven days (Group 1) and 30 days (Group 2) and urine samples were collected at specified time points in the study.

Changes in urinary concentration of the heavy metals were measured by inductively coupled plasma mass spectrometry and compared to the baseline. Also, serum samples were obtained from five individuals in each group and serum electrolytes were measured prior to and after taking the product. Participants in both groups had increased concentrations of heavy metals in the urine with the peak excretion at around day 4. No clinically significant alterations in serum electrolyte levels were seen at either seven or 30 days on ACS. In conclusion, this study demonstrates that the daily use of an activated clinoptilolite suspension represents a potentially safe and effective way to remove toxic heavy metals from the body through increased urinary excretion without removing clinically detrimental amounts of vital electrolytes.[525]

For those most exposed, Zeolite that has been super activated is a required tool for removing maximum levels of radioactive particles from the body at the beginning of a decorporation protocol. When properly used, its most significant benefits occur over the first 30 days. Thereafter, other tools may replace further need of this wonderful product, unless new exposure occurs. Zeolite's properties make it an excellent remover of many radioactive elements, especially 137Cs.[526, 527, 528, 529]

Baking Soda

We make significant amounts of baking soda in our body daily and one function is to aid in the elimination of toxins through the urine. Uranium (238U) is quite stubborn about exiting without a fight and may require not just one elimination channel, but two - the urine as well as the bowels. Baking soda will help to excrete uranium through the kidneys.[530, 531] See next section for more details.

Cell ➔ Blood ➔ Urine/Bile ➔ Bowel Elimination

Melatonin

Melatonin has the distinct advantage above all the other heavy metal chelating agents in that it is also (a) a formidable free radical scavenger as well as (b) the key orchestrator to optimizing cell supplies of glutathione. For this reason, melatonin is considered the single most quintessential tool for antidoting and reversing radiation poisoning.

> *The protective role of exogenous melatonin on U-induced nephrotoxicity was investigated in rats. Animals were given single doses of uranyl acetate dihydrate (UAD) at 5 mg/kg (subcutaneous), melatonin at 10 or 20 mg/kg (intraperitoneal), and UAD (5 mg/kg) plus melatonin (10 or 20 mg/kg), or vehicle (control group). In comparison with the UAD-treated group only, significant beneficial changes were noted in some urinary and serum parameters of rats concurrently exposed to UAD and melatonin. The increase of U excretion after UAD*

administration was accompanied by a significant reduction in the renal content of U when melatonin was given at a dose of 20 mg/kg. Melatonin also reduced the severity of the U-induced histological alterations in kidney. In renal tissue, the activity of the superoxide dismutase (SOD) and the thiobarbituric acid reactive substances (TBARS) levels increased significantly as a result of UAD exposure. Following UAD administration, oxidative stress markers in erythrocytes showed a reduction in SOD activity and an increase in TBARS levels, which were significantly restored by melatonin administration. In plasma, reduced glutathione (GSH) and its oxidized form (GSSG) were also altered in UAD-exposed rats. However, only the GSSG/GSH ratio was restored to control levels after melatonin treatment. Oxidative damage was observed in kidneys. Melatonin administration partially restored these adverse effects. It is concluded that melatonin offers some benefit as a potential agent to treat acute U-induced nephrotoxicity.[532]

And furthermore…

*Melatonin (N-acetyl-5-methoxytryptamine), the chief secretory product of the pineal gland in the brain, is well known for its functional versatility. In hundreds of investigations, melatonin has been documented as a direct free radical scavenger and an indirect antioxidant, as well as an important immunomodulatory agent. The radical scavenging ability of melatonin is believed to work via electron donation to detoxify a variety of reactive oxygen and nitrogen species, including the highly toxic hydroxyl radical. It has long been recognized that the damaging effects of ionizing radiation are brought about by both direct and indirect mechanisms. The direct action produces disruption of sensitive molecules in the cells, whereas the indirect effects (approximately 70%) result from its interaction with water molecules, which results in the production of highly reactive free radicals such as *OH, *H,* *and e(aq)- and their subsequent action on subcellular structures. The hydroxyl radical scavenging ability of melatonin was used as a rationale to determine its radioprotective efficiency. Indeed, the results from many in vitro and in vivo investigations have confirmed that melatonin protects mammalian cells from the toxic effects of ionizing radiation. Furthermore, several clinical reports indicate that melatonin administration, either alone or in combination with traditional radiotherapy, results in a favorable efficacy:toxicity ratio during the treatment of human cancers. This article reviews the literature from laboratory investigations that document the ability of melatonin to scavenge a variety of free radicals (including the hydroxyl radical induced by ionizing radiation) and summarizes the evidence that should be used to design larger translational research-based clinical trials using melatonin as a radioprotector and also in cancer radiotherapy. The potential use of melatonin for protecting individuals from radiation terrorism is also considered.*[533]

Melatonin will help remove many toxic metals (including 238U) from the most internal places within the human body.[534, 535, 536] Just be sure to add in extra amounts of fiber to facilitate Melatonin's job as a quintessential radio-protective agent.

N-Acetyl-Cysteine (NAC)

NAC - This amino acid is an efficient remover of toxic metals via the bowels. For example, radioactive cobalt (60Co), radioactive plutonium (239Pu), and directly and indirectly uranium (238U) all respond to NAC.[537, 538, 539, 540]

Baking Soda

Humans make baking soda in their body daily, 24/7. It is essential for optimal health and wellbeing. One of its least widely known functions is to remove toxic metals from the body.

> *Decorporation therapy is the only known effective method of reducing the radiation dose to persons following accidental internal contamination with transportable radionuclides. Deposits of actinides in bone should be minimized because development of osteosarcoma appears to be related to internal exposure. In contrast with other actinides, such as plutonium or americium where chelating agent treatment is efficient, the therapeutic approaches used for cases of uranium contamination are widely ineffective. This is the first report on in vivo efficacy of a chelating agent, a siderophore analogue code named 3,4,3-LIHOPO, after systematic exposure to natural uranium in the rat. Using the classical antidotal therapy (sodium bicarbonate) for comparison, this ligand has been investigated for its ability to remove uranium from rats after intravenous or intramuscular injection as nitrate. Following an immediate single intramuscular or intravenous injection of 3,4,3-LIHOPO (30 mumol.kg-1) urinary excretion of uranium was greatly enhanced with a corresponding reduction 24 h later in kidney and bone uranium content (to about 20 and 50% of the control rat respectively). Under identical experimental conditions, sodium bicarbonate (640 mumol.kg-1) reduced the uranium content in kidney and bone only to about 90% and 70% of controls respectively, and there was less enhancement of uranium excretion. However, when treatment was delayed by 30 min and administered intraperitoneally, there was no marked difference in retention and excretion of uranium between the two compounds.*[541]

In summary, baking soda is an excellent adjunct (if administered prudently under a physician's instructions) to remove radioactive uranium, and possibly other related heavy metals from the body. Uranium is quite stubborn about exiting without a fight and (in addition to NAC) could require baking soda to speed things up.[542, 543, 544, 545]

The life of the cell is immortal; it is the fluid in which it floats that degenerates.

Alexis Carrel

Chapter Six

The Regeneration Effect™ and Radiation Hormesis

To achieve optimal health, the final phase of handling radiation is to assure that the body is able to regenerate itself. Regeneration can be defined as, "The natural renewal of a structure, as in a lost tissue or part."[546] Or, more precisely it can be defined as, "To generate or produce anew; to replace a (cell or body part) by new growth of tissue; to restore to normal strength or properties."[547] More germane to the consequences of radiation exposure, regeneration may additionally be defined as unscheduled healing or healing that proceeds at an unexpected accelerated speed resulting in a proper or complete healing.

When the human host is stressed or under attack, the resulting damage induces a healing response. Ideally, this healing response possesses the full reserves of a healthy body which brings about normal repair or even unscheduled or accelerated repair beyond what is considered normal. I call this heightened state of repair "The Regeneration Effect™."

Healthy mature, young adults, have the most optimal resistance to radiation exposures, since they are the strongest of any given population. The strongest obviously have something to protect them from radiation poisoning that the weaker members of our population do not have.[548] We must determine what the difference is and then use this to boost our innate resistance.

Fundamentally, regeneration at the cell's core level must start and end by re-establishing the integrity of the cell's high energy gel state (or milieu which reigns supreme over host resistance to radioactive poisoning). The gel state is composed of six essential components:

- ✓ Structured water featuring uniform layers of H_2O molecules because each layer is uniformly polarized (charged), enabling such layers to "stack" on top of each other like colors in a rainbow (scientifically termed Polarized Multilayered Water or PM Water).
- ✓ A broad spectrum of suspended (not dissolved) mineral ions electrically aligned within this PM water.
- ✓ Activating worker bee molecules called "cardinal adsorbents."
- ✓ Select internal cell proteins rich in the amino acid proline and/or "docking sites" (e.g., cardinal sites) uniquely capable of electrically interfacing with 1 through 3 above.
- ✓ Abundant oxygen.
- ✓ Proper pH.[549]

In this chapter, I detail how a diet rich in healing foods (or super foods) is important. I also explain how the other components of The Regeneration Effect™ are important resources for a healthy lifestyle.

The Regeneration Effect™ Has No Known Rival

Each day in every one of your 75 trillion body cells, you will suffer over 100,000 mutations or alterations in your gene center. That equals 7.5 quintillion mutations or injuries (75 with 17 zeros after it) that occur daily and directly where your cells operate the most essential mechanisms for life.[550, 551, 552, 553]

Yet remarkably, any healthy 25-year-old will repair in each and every single cell of his or her body a total of 7,500,000,000,000,000,000 damages to the gene pool daily.[554] This translates into 868,055,555,555,556 corrections each second. Each cell's gene pool is effectively repaired at such speed due to the enzymes previously mentioned in Chapter 4 - HRR and NHEJ. And incredibly, this number does not even include similar injuries in similar numbers that arise in the cell's other essential compartments (i.e., the other organelles and membranes). In all cases, it would appear that the integrity of the above six essential factors governing the cell's high energy gel state provides for the optimal function of these repair enzymes systems.[555] At the gross anatomic level, the recognized father of modern experimental physiology, Claude Bernard (1813-1878), focused predominantly on the cellular milieu, or the internal and external terrain composing and governing the cell. He coined the term strict determinism to describe the method best suited to decipher what physiological results occur when the cellular milieu interacts with stresses of all kinds.

On a daily basis, this optimum system of self-repair vastly exceeds the outcome of any currently known extrinsic therapeutic method or system. This optimum intrinsic repair system has the potential to cure any known natural disease. Indeed, the body's self-healing ability - operating optimally -

is the only real cure for all natural diseases. This system is capable of simple repair, complex repair, sustained repair, local regeneration of cells, and it is even capable of implementing true cell-to-tissue-to-organ regeneration within certain parameters.

The Four Pillars of the Regeneration Effect

The Regeneration Effect™ brings about optimal intrinsic sustained tissue repair from the cell and below cell level on up. Physicians specializing in The Regeneration Effect™ are experts in managing Four Pillars in their patients. The Four Pillars are disciplined detoxification, maximal oxygenation, super-nourishment and select bioenergetics.[556] In mature, young and healthy populations, I have observed that these four operate in excellence. In the long-living cultures[557] from around the world, my research over the past 30 years indicates the same is true.[558, 559, 560, 561, 562] So, the Four Pillars may be seen and understood as the keys to optimal repair as well as to be long-lived.[563] Each of these pillars is discussed below.

Complete Detoxification

The body must remove the wastes it generates and accumulates in order to heal and function properly. Detoxification is the process by which the body removes these wastes. If detoxification mechanisms are operating optimally, the body may function and heal optimally. If body detoxification is compromised, all body healing and function will be compromised as well.

Triggers to Complete Cellular Detoxification – Autophagy

Low levels of radiation that disrupt cell membranes will trigger attempts in tissues to regenerate the damage.[564] Autophagy is the cell's enzymatic system that breaks down damaged components into reusable parts, and then reallocates the parts to more essential processes such as cellular repair or cellular replication. When a cell becomes damaged by ionizing radiation, autophagy "kicks-off" all repair at that cellular level.[565, 566] Internal recycling systems kick into full gear to further break down the damaged pieces into re-usable parts. Unusable residues are simply eliminated. The re-usable reprocessed parts are quickly and efficiently rededicated to patch the cell back up, or to contribute to rebuilding nearby damaged cells. Lastly, these renewed cellular building blocks may enter into the local or systemic pool of spare parts dedicated to new cell replication and complete autophagy.[567]

Rebuilding is dependent upon many circumstances. For example, just enough autophagy, properly guided and stimulated,[568] with sufficient reserves of essential substrates (building blocks) and other essential factors like oxygen, proper pH, and cell water structured in multiple layers with specific electrical charges (dependent upon specific minerals and proline rich peptides derived from the diet),[569] and your body is able to repair itself with great efficiency.[570, 571, 572]

But autophagy can go awry with:

- ✓ Low reserves of the super nutrients
- ✓ Too few antioxidants to protect the integrity of the process
- ✓ Hypoxia (low oxygen levels), a feature of rogue cell regenerative cycles (i.e., cancer)

- ✓ Exposure to new incoming radiation or environmental toxins (xenobiotics)[573]
- ✓ Excessive inflammation

Unhealthy lifestyles contribute to the above conditions. For example, people who live sedentary lifestyles (those who choose to smoke, or people who eat the standard American diet) are at risk. These practices will ensure that low level radiation exposure will speed the onset of chronic degenerative diseases, premature aging or early death.

When ionizing radiation is ongoing, it is important to continually optimize autophagy at the cellular level. The Akizuki Diet supported autophagy via its liberal use of fermented soy (rich in Genistein), sea vegetables (rich in iodine[574] and selenium), cabbage family vegetables (rich in isothiocyanates), and green tea (rich in EGCG).[575, 576, 577, 578, 579] Additionally, the Akizuki Diet is low in calories but rich in nutrients. This also sets up a predisposition for effective cellular repair via autophagy. Autophagy is activated in low calorie periods, especially during fasting.[580]

Beyond the Akizuki Diet, autophagy may be optimally supported by insuring for proper exposure to sunlight (i.e., Vitamin D), use of the herb curcumin, Far Infrared Therapy (FIR), eating raw foods that contain resveratrol and proline rich foods such as whey.[581, 582, 583, 584] Straight-forward dietary guidelines that accomplish much of the above are laid out in the next chapter. You can consume appropriate nutrients by the use of easy-to-make delicious breakfast smoothies the whole family will love.

Inhibitors to Complete Detoxification

Acid wastes poison the pH of cells. Raw foods rich in water and minerals largely correct this problem for people who are eating a proper diet composed of 50% raw foods. Delicious and properly made smoothies easily accomplish this goal along with healthy and uncontaminated cooked foods.

Excessive inflammatory states may accompany the ionization of tissues, which amplifies both the power as well as the number of toxins in the body. Together they must be completely detoxified and tamed. This is accomplished with select herbs, vitamins and minerals.[585, 586, 587] Superior herbal quenchers to inflammation are:

- ✓ Boswellia
- ✓ Cherry extracts
- ✓ Curcumin[588, 589]
- ✓ Green Tea
- ✓ Omega 6 oil extract of Borage Seeds (GLA)
- ✓ Omega 3 oils coming from North Atlantic sourced Cod or Antarctic Krill oils
- ✓ Wasabi[590, 591]
- ✓ Willow bark[592]

For workers in Japan (the "liquidators") exposed to high levels of radiation, this group of superior inflammation quenchers plus highest quality whey and NAC are of paramount importance when attempting to reverse the radiation onslaught. Specially formulated tablets may be taken to efficiently quench most hyper-inflammatory states. See the "Acute Radiation Poisoning" section in the final chapter for full dietary supplement protocols.

Maximum Oxygenation

Our body needs oxygen not only to make energy, but also to regenerate our genetic core when suffering from ROS damage. As previous mentioned, critical function of antioxidant enzymes systems involved with DNA (both SSB and DSB) may require optimal cellular oxygen saturation.[593, 594, 595]

Oxygenation of the body involves intake from the skin, lungs, delivery by blood vessels to cells, and finally special handling of oxygen at the cell level mainly within the cell's mitochondria, where most energy is produced. If oxygenation is sub-optimal due to improper body oxygen saturation or due to inadequate processing by the mitochondria, human tissue regeneration will fail.

The Aikido Diet supplied several items critical to insuring for maximal cellular oxygenation including chlorophyll-rich foods to help rebuild red blood cells (the carriers of oxygen to the cells), green tea, resveratrol, lipoic acid (which collectively may increase the total numbers of mitochondria responsible for burning vast amounts of oxygen efficiently to produce optimal energy), and iodine from sea vegetables to help insure proper thyroid hormone secretion. Proper thyroid hormone secretion is essential for maximal cellular oxygenation.[596, 597]

People of all ages need to insure that their cells get a plentiful supply of oxygen 24/7. This is accomplished by either: (a) physical yoga breathing exercises, (b) undergoing aerobic exercise while keeping your body's pH in an ideal range, (c) exercising while breathing in pure oxygen with a medical device or (d) employing Far Infrared heat (FIR) with oxygen for short durations, and (e) taking nutrients such as the Vitamin B Complex, CoQ10(H), Vinpocetin and alkalinizing agents.[598, 599, 600, 601]

Maximal re-oxygenation is particularly important for folks over 55 who typically have under-saturated tissue oxygenation. [602] This must be corrected to induce cellular regeneration or The Regeneration Effect™. The protocols in the next chapter include easy-to-follow steps for accomplishing maximal oxygen saturation.

After insuring maximal oxygen is reaching your tissues, you need to assure that your cell's mitochondria properly utilize it. Mitochondria are easily damaged or destroyed with ionizing radiation due to the production of ROS and RNS,[603, 604] which is why a top complaint of those poisoned by radiation poisoning is extreme fatigue. In summary, regenerating the number of cellular mitochondria is a top priority after radiation poisoning.

Cell Mitochondrial Regeneration

Perhaps the most common denominator to all chronic degenerative disease is the loss of cellular mitochondria (the cell's engines).[605, 606] Cell mitochondrial regeneration solves the catastrophic loss of cell energy production. Similar to genetic core rebuilding, evidence suggests cell mitochondria must also be properly saturated with oxygen to invigorate antioxidant enzyme repair mechanisms.[607] Additionally, three factors promote the rapid generation of new cellular mitochondria: (a) exercise,[608] (b) calorie restriction[609] and (c) the gene modulator PGC-1 α.[610] The first two increase the levels of PGC-1 α in the body.[611, 612, 613] So, PGC-1 α is the key determinant to generating new cellular mitochondria.

When ionizing radiation destroys cellular mitochondria, the correct strategy to deal with this is to supply all necessary raw materials to optimize the levels and function of PGC-1 α, and then protect them from further harm. This becomes possible by *properly* stimulating a specific cell signaling cascade involving: (a) nitric oxide,[614] (b) SIRT1,[615] and (c) AMPK.[616] Respectively, (a) the amino acids Carnosine, L-arginine and green tea (i.e., EGCG),[617, 618] (b) the polyphenol Resveratrol,[619] (c) lipoic acid and thyroid hormone[620, 621] are known to properly stimulate and support this signaling cascade (providing optimal oxygen saturation is assured through exercise). Again, this may be easily accomplished through select supplementation taken at meal times. Then, by replenishing antioxidants and removing contact with all future radiation (good luck), you can keep your newly regenerated supplies of mitochondria.

There are four counter-indications to regenerating levels of mitochondria arising from exposure to radioactive particles.

First, the radionuclide(s) must be removed before lipoic acid is administered. This is because lipoic acid is an excellent chelator of heavy metals (and therefore possibly metal radionuclides), but may tend to deposit the metals into the cell nucleus.[622] Then, after radionuclides have been eliminated (usually over one to three months, more quickly if hot baths are used with magnetic clays to draw the radioactive particles out of the body, and no new exposure occurs), lipoic acid may be safely included to rebuild optimal levels of cellular mitochondria. However, a unique form of lipoic acid called R-Alpha Lipoic Acid (R-ALA) does not appear to suffer from this problem and may be used from the start.

Second, the amino acid L-arginine should not be given in folks deficient in CoQ10(H). Administering arginine raises nitric oxide levels, which in turn produces excesses of superoxide radical in the absence of CoQ10(H).[623] More importantly, statins tend to make one deficient in CoQ10(H), as does aging.[624] In this case, restoring optimal levels of readily absorbable CoQ10(H) or NAC concomitantly to administering arginine are the simple solutions.[625, 626, 627]

Third, 131-I easily disrupts thyroid function and can lead to permanent health risks.[628, 629, 630, 631, 632, 633] As mentioned above, thyroid hormone plays a huge role in proper mitochondria function.[634] Many folks unknowingly have chronic lower thyroid hormone production (which is oftentimes not sufficiently corrected with synthetic thyroid medications). Low thyroid greatly increases the risk of developing chronic degenerative disease.[635] Unfortunately, conventional medicine has failed to adequately appraise low thyroid conditions, so this only compounds inadequacies in statistical analysis.[636] The good news is that properly designed regenerative programs utilizing optimal supplementation with iodine plus FIR allows you to overcome this.

L-arginine raises inducible nitric oxide (iNO), which in the initial stages of radiation poisoning, may lead to hyper-inflammation. Therefore, mitochondrial regeneration should proceed first with carnosine and green tea as opposed to L-arginine supplementation. Alongside the Carnosine and green tea, the anti-inflammatory program may be initiated (i.e., the "Optimum Radiation Quenching Protocol" section in the next chapter). After all radionuclides have been eliminated, and no further incoming exposure is occurring, L-arginine may be added in to further boost generation of mitochondria. L-lysine should be added into the regimen to balance L-arginine supplementation. Typically, from 1,000mg to 3,000mg daily of L-lysine is given to offset the possibility of L-arginine antagonizing a dormant or ongoing herpes virus infection.

Super Nourishment

Most menu selections in industrialized nations are calorie intense and nutrient poor. Additionally, commercial agricultural practices grow foods today that are more and more deficient in vital nutrients,[637] such as the essential mineral elements.[638, 639] Furthermore, heat-sensitive food factors that spur regenerative healing in human tissues are destroyed by the various methods used to preserve and cook our most popular foods.[640, 641, 642] Therefore, super-nourishment involves obtaining nutrient rich, calorie poor (i.e., high fiber foods) foods grown and prepared under ideal conditions. These ideal conditions are uncontaminated mineral rich soils or waters (rock dust fertilizers for land agriculture or oceanic aquaculture for sea vegetables), plus restricted use of excessive heat to prepare these foods. In this fashion, human tissue regeneration may be started by properly supplying the raw materials required to achieve accelerated or unscheduled healing.[643, 644, 645, 646]

The Akizuki Diet featured several menu items with known properties to induce accelerated healing or regeneration. These included fermented foods, teas and foods high in chlorophyll,[647] foods high in nucleic acids (RNA), teas rich in wound healing agents,[648] and probiotics. For example, sea vegetables are high in both chlorophyll and RNA. Local Japanese land vegetables such as green leafy vegetables like spinach (i.e., horenso-no-gomaae) and members of the cabbage family, are all rich in chlorophyll, Vitamin C, lipoic acid and phenolics like resveratrol, and would have aided healing of the patient's burns from ionizing radiation. It is also highly likely that consumption of vitamin C rich, locally grown (e.g., Hokkaido region, etc.) raw fruits, when available, were also consumed in the Aikido Diet.

At the cell and below cellular level, autophagy leads the effort to self-repair if the proper milieu (local cell environment, i.e., proper pH and oxygenation) and raw materials are available.[649, 650] Specifically, autophagy is heavily involved with coordinating repair of cell membranes and the cell mitochondria and repairing genetic damage to the cell.[651, 652]

Beyond the coordinated efforts of autophagy, we are especially concerned with locking in the gains made through autophagy with optimal antioxidant defenses at the cell membrane, cell mitochondria and cell nucleus.[653] So the diet must supply rich levels of antioxidants on an ongoing basis.

Cell Level Regeneration

Next, The Regeneration Effect™ at the cell level is brought about by crucial building blocks including the optimal gel state.[654, 655] This would include dietary offerings of unique structural proteins. Shark fin soup, which contains proline rich-peptides (P-R-Ps), is one source of unique structural proteins, as is highest quality whey and beef cartilage from range-fed herds that graze in areas free from radioactive fallout. Minerals are crucial, especially colloidal minerals (minerals suspended, not dissolved into liquid). Lightly cooked sea vegetables would be one excellent source. Finally, optimal hydration with mineral rich structured water, as found in organic fruits and vegetables that have been freshly juiced, are ideal to maximize regeneration.[656] Other excellent sources include properly rehydrated sea vegetables[657] bean sprouts, raw green leafy vegetables and select mineral springs.[658,659, 660, 661] Finally, as mentioned previously in Chapter 4, protecting each cell's reserves of HRR and NHEJ from ROS enables regeneration of the genetic core.[662]

Tissue Level Regeneration

Above the cell level, the immune system coordinates all overwhelmed local repair efforts when a major injury is underway in part by precision delivery of super-nutrients which I call colloidal regeneration factors (cRFs).[663, 664] The diet must, therefore, provide for the special needs of the immune system, which include superior growth modulators intrinsic in raw superfoods such as highest quality whey.[665, 666, 667]

Additionally, nutritional modulation of Interferon-gamma will rally this effort, utilizing NAC, zinc and lactoferrin.[668, 669, 670] This support allows the immune system to properly execute the prime repair directive once the local reserves are exhausted, providing that inflammation is under control.[671]

Specifically, consuming algae (rich in nucleic acids and chlorophyll) and select colostrum-rich whey and egg albumin provides transfer factors that are ideal sources of regenerative factors.[672, 673, 674, 675] Some of the best growth determinants come from select algae.[676, 677, 678] Other sources of growth factors come from select dairy proteins.[679] However, all of these sources must be grown or raised in regions not contaminated with radioactive fallout (i.e., the southern Hemisphere or other known locations that are free from anthropogenic radionuclides).

Organ Level Regeneration

To regenerate organs, optimal hormonal functions are required, such as optimal thyroid and growth hormone levels and liver function.[680, 681, 682, 683] The proline rich peptides in whey appear to be important to help initiate stem cell repair systems.[684] Other excellent sources of growth factors come from freeze-dried animal glandular extracts.[685, 686, 687]

In review, the following list of natural tools helps generate and sustain regenerative effects after exposure to anthropogenic radiation. The nutrients contained in the following foods and tools may likely enable the host to accelerate repair after cellular damage from ionizing radiation:

- ✓ High raw food diet, fresh organic juices, plus thyroid medication, potassium, table salt restriction, iodine, low-dose aspirin and detoxification[688, 689, 690]
- ✓ Milk thistle (silymarin)[691]

- ✓ Aloe[692]
- ✓ Green Tea[693]
- ✓ Whey[694, 695]
- ✓ Chlorella[696, 697]
- ✓ Spirulina (phycocyanin)[698, 699, 700, 701]
- ✓ Colloidal Regeneration Factors (cRFs™)[702, 703, 704, 705, 706, 707]
- ✓ Chlorophyll[708]
- ✓ Probiotics[709, 710, 711]

The next chapter highlights easy-to-use supplementation protocols to help accomplish the above.

Bioenergetics

Finally, select bioenergetics are required to establish a lasting Regeneration Effect. Bioenergetics includes the principles of "mind-over-matter" as well as the power of prayer, and also extends into music or sound therapy, light therapy, heat therapy, magnetic therapy, etc. For example, having a sense of humor and using laughter to move through stressful situations (i.e., knowing you live in zones exposed to radiation) greatly influences your ability to heal properly.[712]

Music or sound therapy is an emerging science that may have powerful effects on human tissue repair.[713] In fact, "BioAcoustical Profiling" often pegs emotional fixations or mental intention of the individual to their health issues.[714] This relaxing even soothing technology can easily be employed in the convenience of your own home.

Also for the home setting, convenient bed pads that possess select magnetic fields will remove stress and greatly enhance deep sleep as well as raise tissue oxygen levels.[715, 716, ,717, 718, 719] Both of these techniques may help speed healing.

In the medical setting, Bioenergetics includes low voltage stimulation (via electrical acupuncture) and laser acupuncture.

One of the latest discoveries in bioenergetic medicine involves vitagenes. Vitagenes are a group of genes that preserve and repair essential cellular components such as DNA and RNA. They repair genetic damage. Heat therapy is a very accessible bioenergetic tool, and Far Infrared Therapy (FIR) or hot baths may easily support and elicit the vitagene regenerative response.[720] Vitagenes are especially supported with the simultaneous use of the amino acids Acetyl-L-Carnitine (ALCAR) and Carnosine.[721]

Finally, select homeopathic remedies are known to be beneficial in lessening the symptoms and pathology of radiation poisoning. More on this in later editions.

Misconceptions About Radiation Hormesis – Russian Roulette or Regenerative Aikido?

In biology, hormesis means a small amount of a substance will tend to stimulate, while a larger amount of that substance will tend to inhibit. Unfortunately, this definition cannot be applied to ionizing radiation. We know from the Petkau Effect that small doses of radiation over long timeframes causes more damage than high doses of radiation over a shorter time period, so that's one strike.

Furthermore, bystander effects appear contrarian to the theory of radiation hormesis. Both the Petkau Effect and bystander effect arise from units of host absorbed radiation called "radiation absorbed dose" (rad) or "Gray" units (Gy). One (1) Gy unit equals 100 rad. It is known that an identical low dose rate (LDR) of tissue radiation may induce bystander effects that paradoxically either inhibit *or* stimulate tissues. The fact that the low dose has the potential to inhibit is contrarian to the principle of hormesis, so strike two. Additionally, a single low dose of radiation (i.e., < 2 rad) may be too low to invoke tissue repair reactions. So without repair systems activated, low doses may become more lethal to cells than "slightly higher" doses (i.e., > 2 rad). That's strike three. Next, Sgouros, et al showed that lower doses of radiation, two (2) rad per hour, weakened tissue resistance to follow-on radiation five (5) times *more* than 100 rad per hour! [722, 723] That's strike four against the theory of radiation hormesis

Therefore, beneficial immune responses from low dose radiation (erroneously ascribed to hormesis) would be better attributed to host resistance (i.e., activation of select antioxidants and repair systems).[724, 725] Dynamics of host resistance confronting radiation is best deciphered by Strict Determinism. Strict Determinism is a method that deciphers physiological causes and effects.

As previously mentioned, the father of modern experimental physiology was Claude Bernard, who defined for the first time how experimentation was required to reveal theories relevant to physiology (i.e., working hypothesis), as well as to eventually prove such theories (working hypothesis which may eventually become a law of physiology). Strict Determinism was the core principle he saw underlying all physiology, which would always reveal itself during the course of painstaking, repeated, identical, experimentation. In a nut shell, the resilience of the cell, tissue, organ or animal matters most, not the parameters or design of the experiment.

Specifically, Strict Determinism states, "Under precisely controlled experimental conditions, the test animal does as it damn well pleases." Why do some test animals die and others live when exposed to a given amount of radiation over exact time frames? The collective cell physiology of the animals determined the outcome of the experiments - their resistance factors, strengths and weaknesses, *not* the external parameters of the experiment. Bernard concluded that, "The fixity of the internal environment is the condition for free life."[726] Or put into plain English, "The resilience of the cellular milieu is the prerequisite for living disease-free."

So what about advocates of radiation hormesis? What evidence do they put forward to make the case for beneficial effects from man-made radiation? In essence, in select subpopulations (i.e., the affluent and otherwise healthy ~20 to 50 year olds), people may possess the innate strength to repair ionizing radiation over other sub-groups. There are examples in the authoritative literature suggesting that within narrow parameters of low levels of radiation exposure, nondestructive or even temporary beneficial effects may be realized in the young and healthy. [727, 728, 729, 730] But these examples are deciphered according to Strict Determinism, and cannot be deciphered by the theory of radiation hormesis.[731]

Advocates of radiation hormesis also cite mineral rich hot springs which are known to emit low level radiation from a naturally occurring radioisotope called radon.[732] There are no studies to date that make comparisons between anthropogenic and natural radioisotopes relating to beneficial effects. Yet, unsubstantiated comparisons are still drawn. This is the classic mistake of scientists when they leave behind common sense; that is, confusing similar things as identical things.

For example, it is true that the hot springs in Attica, Lesvos and Ikaria, Greece, and in the Misasa Hot Springs

District of Japan are renown for spontaneous healings arising from proper use of the therapeutic waters.[733, 734, 735] These hot springs are typically used to provide short-term radon exposures to folks, and with levels of radon exposure that have been naturally encountered by human beings for millennia. However, harmful sequelae appears to be associated with: (a) longer exposure periods, as well as to (b) higher levels of mixed radioactive contaminants (i.e., 238U plus radon).[736, 737]

I would like to further illustrate that the emerging science of radiation hormesis ignores the original principle of experimental physiology, which is Bernard's "Strict Determinism." If we consider what happens to our skin when we get sunburned as a teenager, the redness passes by in a day or two as the skin flakes off and is simply replaced with new pink baby skin. The radiation occurred naturally from the sun, not from absorbed hot particles impregnated into the skin. Again, similar things in physiology are never identical. The sun's radiation killed the skin cells prematurely, and they fell off. The repair system was triggered due to the sensory feedback systems of the host. The sun's UV light induced production of Vitamin D which spurs autophagy. These feedback systems work regardless of the induced stress, and are not exclusive to radiation. A simple scrape would have triggered the identical sensory feedback system to initiate repair minus the extra Vitamin D.

Now consider what happens with tiny "hot spots" of internal radioactivity - it causes lethal ionizing internal sunburns 24/7 within tiny, highly localized areas of our tissues. This creates a localized alarm reaction, which inevitably turns up the mechanisms of autophagy and other mechanisms of repair (such as Nrf2, PGC-1α, HRR, NHEJ, etc…), in the strong and healthy.[738, 739, 740, 741] If the hot particle can be eliminated, and the repair system of the host is intact, repair may result. If the hot particles remain steadfast, an endless cycle of damage and attempts at repair will ensue. Two steps backward in terms of damage, and at best two steps forward in terms of repair. No net gain or loss until the repair system loses its "fixity."

In those with weaker resistance, or in those who are dosed excessively, nothing can be done to defeat the overwhelming physics of ionizing radiation because their fixity has been degenerated or destroyed. In all of these varying situations, Strict Determinism is our vantage point to decipher the conditions for living disease-free. Once deciphered, we just have to bolster and/or regenerate the resilience to the intracellular milieu.

Within this setting of those with weaker resistance or those who are dosed excessively, prevention, antidoting with antioxidants, consuming superfoods rich in growth factors, and elimination of all offending toxins is required to establish proper healing. Utilizing Strict Determinism, we observe that these four galvanize the weaker resilience of the host (i.e., galvanize the fixity of the host's internal cellular environment); however, if the resilience of the host cannot be restored, the individual may still become seriously ill or die.

When the local tissue response to heal is overwhelmed, systemic systems of repair must come online to keep up with the intensity of internal repair.[742] Then, glandular secretions of hormones and growth factors, immune cell mediators and stem cell maturation mechanisms jump into action.[743, 744, 745] Orchestrating this systemic mobilization to insure that the intensity of repair exceeds the intensity of the internal ionizing damage are the bioenergetics of epigenesis and cell-to-cell signaling.[746, 747, 748]

In review, the Regeneration Effect is the optimal fixity possible for the human physiology. This optimal fixity is comprised of

Four Pillars which define, restore and maintain the resilience of the host: (a) cellular, tissue and organ detoxification, (b) full oxygen saturation, (c) super-nourishment to all tissues, and (d) timely, clear and complete cell-to-cell, cell-to-tissue, tissue-to-organ signaling (proper physiological communications). Over the past five-thousand years, no less than 20, independent, long-living and extremely healthy subpopulations teased-out, honed, perfected and proved the methods of the Four Pillars, which always lead to The Regeneration Effect™ Additionally, hundreds of tissue experiments as well as thousands of animal experiments confirm the methods to the Four Pillars as painstakingly worked out via simple trial and error by our healthiest forefathers.[749, 750, 751, 752, 753, 754]

Optimal management of The Regeneration Effect™ is likely the best method to successfully play regenerative aikido with "radiation." Anything less will lead to cellular Russian roulette. Ionizing radiation is not just akin to playing with fire, but playing simultaneously with multiple raging infernos at the cell, tissue and organ levels. Before venturing any further into the suppositions of radiation hormesis, remember that there is no safe level of anthropogenic radiation exposure.[755, 756] By these set of facts, we may dismiss the notion of radiation hormesis, and start discussing how to accelerate host repair systems in light of the Fukushima Catastrophe.

If we must play regenerative aikido with ionizing radiation, let us do it with the Four Pillars, which is the methodology to regenerative medicine.

Conclusion

The information in this chapter helps you understand why some people and animals temporarily survive and thrive after radiation exposure. It has also discussed the cellular impact of various nutrients you can use to combat the biophysical effects of radiation poisoning at the cellular level and below. Utilizing Strict Determinism, it all boils down to:

1. The prior cumulative stresses already present in the host.
2. The antioxidant capacity and potential (substrate reserves) of tissues.
3. The radioactive dosage levels and steady or interrupted streams of free-radical formation (length of exposure).
4. The elimination capacity and efficiency of the host for radioactive toxic particle elimination.
5. The capacity of the host to repair at the below cell, cell, tissue and organ level, as reflected in the eight factors (after Petkau, Ling and Tennant).[757, 758, 759]

From the viewpoint of radiation biophysics and how it impacts host resistance, it all boils down to:

- ✓ The specific radioactive particle involved (i.e., what kind of ionizing radiation does it emit, and what other non-ionizing toxic effects the particular heavy metal may possess).
- ✓ Does the ionizing radiation overwhelm the lipid antioxidant defenses of the host's tissues?
- ✓ Does the ionizing radiation overwhelm normal oxygen utilization of the cell?
- ✓ Does the ionizing radiation overwhelm the buffering capacity of the cell and disrupt the cell's pH profile?
- ✓ Does the ionizing radiation disrupt the cell's internal structured water (i.e., structured alkaline water)?[760]

- ✓ Does the ionizing radiation disrupt the normal spectrum or function of mineral elements in the cell?
- ✓ Does the ionizing radiation disrupt the special proline-rich-peptides that are essential to the proper function of structured alkaline water and mineral elements within the cells?
- ✓ Is the Phase Angle of the body damaged by the ionizing radiation?
- ✓ And finally, are the negative millivolts of the cell and tissues disrupted by the ionizing radiation?

The answer to each of the above questions is, of course, yes, meaning that ionizing radiation has a negative effect on the body's resistance and overall health. This is the antithesis of The Regeneration Effect™.

It is easier now to gain proper perspective when hearing official statements regarding exposure levels to radiation in times of a nuclear fallout crisis. Officials and scientists who downplay man-made, low level anthropogenic radiation arising from nuclear power plant accidents by characterizing them as: "normal background radiation levels," "permissible radiation levels" or "potentially beneficial" due to the phenomenon of "hormesis," do the general public a grave injustice. Until they circumspect the above eight essential factors that govern cell physiology, plus fully acknowledge the Petkau Effect, the bystander effect, and the real epidemiological data documented by Mangano, Wing, Busby and Yablokov, they stand upon conjectural data points largely out of context.[761, 762, 763, 764, 765]

The final chapter will take into account the multi-stage: cell-to-cell, cell-to-tissue, tissue-to-tissue, tissue-to-organ repair mechanisms plus the above eight factors to formulate the best protocols utilizing the principles of Applied Colloidal Therapeutics.™ In a simple and straightforward format, these protocols (designed to both help recover from and prevent further damage from radiation poisoning), will include individualizing all recommendations based upon weight, and according to any budgetary constraints.

Part III

Protecting Your Family

From this point forward, the periodical spikes in our food chain's cycles of bioaccumulation and biomagnification are likely to be deceptively helter-skelter. For example, after the initial fallout contaminates select regional soils across North America, certain soils rich in clay content will be excellent absorbers and retainers of those radioactive particles for a period of time. But gradually after enough rainfall, flooding or forest fires, those particles are eventually re-liberated to freely "float up" the food chain.[766]

Furthermore, highly contaminated soils, waters or fauna are now being exported regionally to unsuspecting consumers. For example, meats, milk, rice or soy grown in Japan,[767, 768] or seaweeds grown and harvested from regions most proximal to the fallout (i.e., Japan's territorial waters, plus eastern China's and South Korea's near coastal waters),[769, 770, 771] will likely threaten millions of unsuspecting consumers globally as time rolls on. Not even the widely used food grade algae products (i.e., chlorella and spirulina) grown in Japan or Taiwan or even Hawaii will escape unscathed. This is the exact pattern we saw after the Chernobyl Catastrophe.[772]

We and our children are at the top of the food chain. So, as the consequences of the local, regional and global migration of Fukushima fallout rolls out, produce grown and cattle raised on such soils become a long-term lethal threat.[773, 774] For example, on July 8th, 2011, the Greater Los Angeles Basin exhibited ongoing excessive levels of radiation. Within this region, a local farmers market was found selling peaches inundated with radioactive particles destined to incessantly ionize the tissues of anyone unsuspectingly eating the fruit. Then later on July 19th, ongoing radioactive particles were being continuously collected in air filters inside buildings over this same area.[775]

The deceptively helter-skelter radionuclide migration, bio-accumulation and biomagnification over weeks, months, years and even decades requires our utmost attention. A most disturbing example pertinent to this discussion was recently documented by nuclear engineering researchers at UC Berkeley. They began been monitoring foods (like milk) produced in the greater San Francisco area when the Fukushima Daiichi accident first occurred.

One of the milk samples revealed that as of August 22nd, 2011, 134Cs was detected at 0.047 Bq/L, and 137Cs at 0.052 Bq/L; yet on September 12th, 2011, these radionuclide levels rose - for 134Cs to 0.55 Bq/L and for 137Cs to 0.059 Bq/L. And as of September 29th, 2011, most alarmingly, milk samples revealed that 134Cs had escalated to 0.080 Bq/L and 137Cs to 0.101 Bq/L. This last sample was more than *160% above the EPA's Maximum Contaminant Level (MCL)*.[776, 777] This is a clear example of bioaccumulation and biomagnification starting in the food supply, and suggests that much worse is yet to come. These radionuclides will inevitably work their way into our meats, cheeses and fertilizers.

I favored above the EPA's more conservative MCL measuring scale (which applies to drinking water) to gauge health risk because the *1500 times more excessive* FDA's derived intervention levels (DIL) limits (which apply to milk) is simply out to lunch - as previously noted in the latter half of Chapter 2. Why? Well, for the same reason we should discredit the

ICRP's methodology - the DIL calculations do not take into account the real-life impact of low dose radiation upon children eating at the top of the food chain. Just as the ICRP measuring scale, DIL utilizes mathematical projections based on science that stands apart from true, real-life health consequences upon human populations receiving fallout from nuclear accidents.[778]

For example, beyond the extended time period it takes a normal body to remove radionuclides when adsorbed deeply into the bone, there is the compounding influence of bioaccumulation, biomagnification and the long-term impact of epigenetic (internal cell genetic signaling) miscommunications part and parcel to the bystander effect.[779, 780, 781, 782, 783,784] Essentially, FDA's DIL would have us believe that if our kids drink milk containing one-hundred times less radionuclide levels than levels found within the previous month's milk, our kids will be somehow miraculously protected! And they call this science?

Obviously our kids are at greatest risk to these kinds of repetitive and cumulative exposures. Therefore, parents should consider minimizing or eliminated milk products as specified next in Chapter 7. There are plenty of uncontaminated and delicious milk substitutes (like calcium-rich almond milk) that will offer healthier alternatives.

We must now remain ever vigilant to this cumulative ionizing radiation. For it is destined to set in motion a never-ending, ubiquitous and most difficult to detect free radical mutational onslaught throughout Japan's and North America's food chain. The "never-ending" aspect is profoundly transgenerational, and "ubiquitous" because this risk applies to all life forms on planet earth. For this reason I dedicate this final chapter to practical radioprotection for both the short term and long term.

*Please note that the guidelines provided in my book are not intended to replace the medical advice of your doctor, or to be construed as medical advice or treatment. A qualified holistic physician familiar with radioprotective therapeutics may largely agree and order their patients to follow the guidelines presented in *Fukushima Meltdown & Modern Radiation: Protecting Ourselves and Our Future Generations*. But you should not expect all physicians to prescribe a medical treatment plan consistent with the guidelines provided in this book.

In considering and evaluating the procedures, steps, and protocols provided in *Fukushima Meltdown & Modern Radiation,* note that for the reader they are intended to exclusively serve as educational facts, guidelines and principles known to be scientifically consistent with successful methods in radio-protection. If you decide to implement any of these protocols into your dietary, please first consult with a qualified holistic physician familiar with radioprotective therapeutics in order to avoid any potential adverse events that may pertain to your specific state of health. Note that this disclaimer applies to the entire content in Parts II and III, and especially to all asterisks appearing in the text.

Our belief at the beginning of a doubtful undertaking is the one thing that assures the successful outcome of any venture.

William James

Chapter Seven

Recovering Your Health

The purpose of this chapter is to provide specific guidance and empowerment for protecting your health in the face of this ongoing threat. By being pro-active, we can minimize or even eliminate the insidious risks from radioactive fallout. You will find instructions on the types of foods to minimize or avoid and potential antidotes if you cannot avoid them.[785]

Who Is Most at Risk?

The following people should strongly consider implementing long-term measures to counteract the broad spectrum of health risks from anthropogenic radiation exposures. The checklist below is a convenient way to estimate the known risks associated with ionizing radiation. Circle each checkmark that applies to you. Count your checkmarks and write the total number in the space provided below:[786, 787]

- ✓ Folks in the United States who reside in areas of high precipitation during the immediate four weeks (and possibly up to 16 weeks) after March 18th.[788, 789]
- ✓ Folks living in the southern half of Alaska, all of Hawaii and the entire west coast of the United States.

- ✓ Recovered cancer patients who have undergone radioablative therapy or nuclear medicine treatments (i.e., received radioactive iodine treatment for a hyperactive thyroid gland).
- ✓ Folks living up to 100 miles downwind of an operational nuclear power plant.[790, 791, 792, 793]
- ✓ Babies, infants and toddlers living within radiation risk zones (the very young are 10 times more sensitive to radioactive exposure than healthy adults).[794, 795, 796, 797]
- ✓ Folks with immune compromise (such as HIV positive individuals or organ transplant recipients or advanced cancer patients).
- ✓ Folks with neurological pathologies.
- ✓ Women with a history of breast cancer.
- ✓ The elderly.
- ✓ Smokers.
- ✓ Folks drinking water containing radon or residing in living quarters perched above radon rich deposits.
- ✓ Hospital workers who specialize in nuclear medicine or who operate ionizing diagnostic equipment such as CAT Scans.
- ✓ Radiology technicians.
- ✓ Chiropractic staff who use X-Ray equipment.
- ✓ Dental staff who use X-Ray equipment.
- ✓ Veterinary staff who use X-Ray equipment.
- ✓ Nuclear industry workers.

- ✓ Military personnel who have been exposed to depleted uranium.
- ✓ Flight attendants and flight crews.
- ✓ All other employees in industry who must utilize X-Ray imaging devices such as TSA officers.
- ✓ Folks residing in Japan, Taiwan, the eastern coastal regions of China, South Korea and Russia who find themselves living in regions contaminated with radioactivity ≥4 kBq/m^2.[798, 799, 800]
- ✓ Folks living in regions exhibiting ≥ 50 Bq/Kg of soil contamination with 137Cs.[801]
- ✓ Anyone with cumulative radiation levels ≥15 Bq/kg bodyweight (BW) and any child with levels ≥5 Bq/kg BW.[802, 803]
- ✓ Families and future children of the liquidators of the Fukushima Catastrophe.[804]

- ✓ Total Check Marks circled: ______
  For educational purposes only, use this number for later reference under the section in this chapter pertaining to individual protection protocols.

Overview of Prevention Measures

Below is a list of the basic prevention measures that everyone should review. Because radiation exposure affects all aspects of our lives, it is important to protect our air, water and food.

- ✓ Drinking water - Use home Charcoal/RO Water Filtration systems, or the cheaper alternatives such as Zero Water® pitcher filtration
- ✓ Bathing water - Use Charcoal/Vitamin C or Zeolite shower heads for showering
- ✓ Home Air - HEPA Air Filtration for home air conditioning and heating units
- ✓ Car Air - Frequently change auto air conditioner filters
- ✓ Fresh Fruits and Vegetables - Wash/soak vegetables and fruits in a sink with 2 tablespoons baking soda or ¼ cup magnetic clay per sinkful of water for 10 minutes before using
- ✓ Rain Exposure - Avoid getting rained on whenever possible
- ✓ House Cleaning - When mopping, use wet mops so that radioactive particles are trapped and then washed away, as opposed to just being stirred back up in the air with dry mopping
- ✓ Clothing - Hang coats on hangers outside (garage, porch, etc…)

Overview of Dietary Guidelines

The first order of business in developing a long-term strategy to combat radiation poisoning is to prevent up front exposure as much as possible. What we eat over the long haul is of critical importance in this regard. The following tables provide dietary guidance for minimizing foods that over time have the potential to be unsuspected and repeated sources of new radionuclide contamination due to the insidious vicissitudes of bioaccumulation and biomagnification.

Proteins

Emphasize	**Minimize**
Eating Low on the food chain. Nuts, nut butters and nut milks, seeds and seed butter (tahini), beans (soy – tofu, tempeh, soy sausage, vege-burgers), peas, whole grains, organic fruits and organic vegetables. Aged beef still ok until dated as slaughtered before March 17th, 2011 or if from regions in the world with no known fallout risk	Red Meat. All red meat products slaughtered after March 17th, 2011 until at least March 2012 when bioaccumulation studies become available.
Wild (non-farmed) North Atlantic sea foods. Emphasize North Atlantic sea fish: Atlantic Cod, Atlantic Pollock, Blue Whiting and Red Hake; Atlantic Haddock; Atlantic Herring; Atlantic Mackerel; Atlantic Salmon; Atlantic Tuna – North Atlantic Bluefin, Yellowfin and Longfin albacore; Atlantic Yellowtail; Black Sea Bass; Monkfish (Angler Fish).	North Pacific Seafood. *Possible Alternatives:* When available, buy frozen or prepared North East Pacific seafood collected prior to March 17th, 2011. The saga of North Pacific seafood bioaccumulation of radioactive toxins will continue now for many years to come.

Proteins Continued.

Emphasize	Minimize
Use egg replacement, or while preparing eggs, use small amounts (pinch) of Calcium Bentonite if prolonged cooking is to be employed. Or, use pectin on low heat, with short cooking time. Thoroughly mix in pectin during dish preparation to help chelate out possible radionuclides.	Poultry products prepared after March 17th, 2011. Especially avoid eggs (even range-fed or organic chicken eggs), unless from regions in North America with no known fallout risk (i.e., the dry, arid regions, such as Mexico, Arizona, New Mexico, Nevada, many parts of Utah (excluding SLC and lowlands receiving rainwater from mountains, south Florida, Maine).
Seafood from Australia, New Zealand, and South America, excluding Gulf of Mexico.	Gulf of Mexico Seafood Avoid these until residues of the British Petroleum oil spill of 2010 are known to have dissipated (i.e., shrimp).

Dairy Products

Emphasize	**Minimize**
Organic coconut milk, coconut yogurt, coconut butter, coconut ice creams, coconut water, hemp butter. Organic It's Better Than Milk®, soy milk, soy ice creams, soy yogurt, soy cheeses, tofu, tempeh, Tofutti ice cream. Organic whole rice milk, rice yogurt, rice ice creams; organic whole oat milk. Organic hemp milk, hemp ice cream, hemp butter; organic almond milk, almond yogurts, almond ice cream; organic hazelnut milk. Organic (non-GMO) "trans-fat-free" margarines. Emphasize two-year aged cheeses (make your home-made pizza with hard, aged cheeses like Romano, parmesan, kasseri, etc…, not mozzarella). Where available, buy dairy products from the So. Hemisphere (i.e., New Zealand, S. America) or select areas not affected by Chernobyl (i.e., western half of France, Spain, Portugal, Sicilia, Sardegna, South Italy).	Fresh dairy products (milk, yogurt, ice cream, BUTTER). *Possible Alternatives:* Use small amounts of calcium bentonite or pectin or calcium alginate to chelate out radionuclides in fresh local dairy products (i.e., 1/8th teaspoon per cup of dairy or dairy milk shake). Buy low sugar-organic yogurt with fruit already blended in (rich in pectin) or mix fresh fruit puree yourself into your ice creams, kefir, sour buttermilk, etc… to help prevent ingestion of radionuclides while you make the dairy even more nutritious. Sour cream, cream cheese and butter could separately be blended with tasteless calcium bentonite (in fine powder form) in a seamless fashion, although it would be a "gooey" stirring process – 1/8th teaspoon per cup.

Fruits, Vegetables and Beverages

Emphasize	**Minimize**
Filtered water; ALL-NATURAL sodas (Hansen's®, Izze®, natural ginger ale, natural root beer, birch beer, etc…). Organic coffee from S. America. Organic green tea – from S. Hemisphere. Organic ginger tea – from India. Organic black tea – from India. Organic white tea – from S. Hemisphere. Organic vegetable juices. Organic (no sugar added) fruit juices (*avoid* juices containing strawberries and other low-to-ground fruits).	Wild grown mushrooms and berries (especially strawberries). Teas, rice, beef and pork from Japan and Eastern China and South Korea.
Organic hot house or hydroponic organic vegetables and fruits protected by over-hanging water-proof barriers are ideal.	Genetically engineered (GE) or gene modified organisms (GMO) (i.e., non-organic fruits and vegetables), especially canola oil and corn oil and all hydrogenated oils and trans-fats.

Fruits, Vegetables and Beverages Continued

Emphasize	Minimize
100% sugar-free jams, especially organic grape, organic apricot, organic marmalade and organic cherry. 100% sugar-free organic apple sauce, pear sauce, plum sauce, etc… 100% maple syrup (organic preferred). Raw coconut tree sap (i.e., Coconut Secret®). Agave syrup, guava syrup. FOS (fructooligosaccharides); ribose. Xylitol, chicory root (i.e., Just Like Sugar®), or organic erythritol (fermented cane juice, i.e., Organic Zero®); or stevia (i.e., Truvia®). Raw honey if collected prior to March 20th or if known to be collected from uncontaminated regions (e.g., desert). Sorghum or black molasses. May use cinnamon, cardamom, natural vanilla, anise, chocolate, carob or other organic flavors or seasonings.	Refined sugar, candies and artificial sweeteners such as aspartame, or high fructose corn syrup. Irradiated spices and seasonings. Any foods (i.e., honey or spices) imported from Belarus, Ukraine and lower western Russia. Avoid like the plague honey collected from regions laced with fallout, as well as refined sugar for reasons beyond the subject of this book.

Fruits, Vegetables and Beverages Continued

Emphasize	Minimize
Algae and sea vegetable products grown in the southern hemisphere or in known uncontaminated regions (i.e., North Atlantic bladderwort, or for products grown or harvested proximal to the Indian and Antarctic Oceans).	Algae products (i.e., spirulina, seaweeds, chlorella) grown in Hawaii, or the west coast of the United States (i.e., Upper Klamath Lake), or in Japan, Taiwan[805] or from regions proximal to the east coast of China and Korea.

Note that strawberries and mushrooms are notorious accumulators of radionuclides from fallout.[806, 807] In fact, present day Nagasaki still produces mushrooms with significant amounts of radionuclides, arguably from the atomic bomb detonation of 1945 coupled to ongoing nuclear power plant releases.[808] The alarming aspect is the long-term devastating impact on birth defects by bioaccumulation of radionuclides throughout the food chain.[809]

I do not give the algae recommendations lightly. Seaweeds and algae are among the most efficient bioaccumulators of radioactive particles known.[810, 811, 812, 813, 814, 815] Located in south central Oregon, Upper Klamath Lake (elevation 4,147 feet), is seven miles long. At many parts along the lake, it is only 8 to 10 feet deep. The lakebed is approximately 30 feet thick with wonderful mineral sediment that normally makes the indigenous food grade algae there (*Aphanizomenon flos*-aquae or *AFA*) one of the greatest super foods on the planet.

However, since western North America (stretching from Alaska down to southern California), has received significant and harmful levels of radionuclides, it is unlikely this lakebed has escaped receiving significant and harmful levels of these radionuclides.[816, 817, 818] Additionally, Upper Klamath Lake receives much of the rain run-off from the nearby mountain range (elevation just over 7,000 feet), where additional radionuclide particles are bound to have landed, destined sooner or later for downstream migration.[819] This regional topography is a perfect example of how bioaccumulation starts and biomagnifies up the food chain.[820]

I would also expect mutations to occur in single-celled organisms as time goes on. If this turns out to be true, these mutations may go ugly.[821] I have written two books on the health properties to *AFA,* including one best-seller, and simply love the product when properly produced.[822, 823] My entire family has been on *AFA* now for over 17 years, and until comprehensive and exhaustive follow-up testing is instituted, I am only consuming *AFA* from the pre-2011 harvest.

Being so personally invested in Upper Klamath Lake's super food *AFA,* I traveled down to the region in early August 2011 to collect car air filter samples in order to screen for possible signs of a local fallout contamination. I collected seven used car and truck air filters from vehicles resident in or near the city of Klamath Falls. Results for these seven air filters have come back negative, meaning no hot particles associated from the Fukushima Catastrophe were detected at this time.[824] The next step is to take local soil samples and send these off for analysis. My current working theory is that over time *AFA* will collect significant amounts of radionuclides from the Fukushima Catastrophe, but as of this writing, the data is inconclusive.

The algae harvesting industry in Upper Klamath Lake is well-known for its meticulous testing procedures for quality control. Let them now add in highly sensitive testing for radionuclides.

The problem is this - what if radionuclides are detected in the harvested product as I expect will occur in the 2011 harvests and those going forward? Would those who have strong ties to the super food release the data to the general public? I know some of the company officials, and these folks are of the highest integrity. But with so much investment at stake, and so many folks on the product under MLM businesses, only time will tell.

The process of bioaccumulation into *AFA* will unfold both near term and long term. There will be days in any given year when the radionuclide content will be low or undetectable.

But during blooms, there is a high probability that on select days of harvest, the radionuclide content could be unacceptably high, such as after new rainfall. So, I am sticking to my recommendation unless and until all data confirms to the contrary. Enough said.

Sample Menu Items

The following daily programs are arranged according to body weight, budgetary concerns and then special needs. Also, this chapter defines context, both in terms of who should consider short- and long-term radioprotective measures. And, I provide information on how others have used these antidotes to protect themselves in the past.

Dietary Suggestions - Wherever possible, follow the rules for eating low on the food chain and washing or decontaminating foods and liquids accordingly. One or more smoothies daily are highly recommended, plus liberal use of properly made Miso soup one or more times weekly, lightly steamed cabbage family vegetables, broccoli sprouts, homemade sauerkraut, home-made coleslaw without eggs, and organic fruits (pre-washed) daily (excluding strawberries from contaminated zones), yogurt with live probiotics made with select nut milks, grain milks or bean milks sweetened with allowable sweeteners and raw organic fruit puree.

Smoothies - Arguably, the easiest way to deal with the radiation crisis is to drink your way through it! By using pre-mix smoothie powders, or making your own, body radiation may be effectively reduced and eliminated. Furthermore, with additional supplementation, it may be possible to reverse much of the damage by enhancing internal repair systems. Smoothies can be of two varieties - fruit based recipes and (dairy-free) milk-based recipes.

Smoothies are best made in a super blender with either:

- ✓ Select, unsweetened milk of choice (It's Better Than Milk® or soy milk if no allergy is present, coconut milk, hemp milk, almond milk, hazelnut milk, rice milk), or coconut water.
- ✓ As an all-fruit sorbet (i.e., Orange Julius - with blood red oranges or nectarines, or grapes, apples, pears, mangos, bananas, peaches, blueberries, etc... but AVOID strawberries, raspberries, blackberries and black raspberries unless grown in uncontaminated soils).

Allowable sweeteners are: organic maple syrup; raw coconut tree sap (i.e., Coconut Secret®); agave syrup, guava syrup; FOS (fructooligosaccharides); ribose; xylitol, mannose or manitol, chicory root (i.e., Just Like Sugar®), or organic erythritol (fermented cane juice, i.e., Organic Zero®); or stevia (i.e., Truvia®); raw honey only if from uncontaminated regions; whole grain malt syrup (i.e., barely malt syrup), or sorghum or black molasses. You may use cinnamon, cardamom, natural vanilla, anise, chocolate, carob, or other organic flavors or seasonings as desired. For a more rich taste, add in ½ banana per smoothie.

One or two delicious tasting smoothies per day is all it takes. See below for recipes.

Anytime Antioxidant Smoothie – AA Smoothie **(makes 10 – 12 ounces):***

<u>Preferred Liquids</u> - 1 cup all-natural vanilla or chocolate flavored organic nut, legume or grain milk of choice, all rich in Vit. B Complex, Vit. E Complex, tocotrienols and phytates from their bran and germ (featuring **antioxidants and**

radionuclide elimination);[825] blended together with **specially formulated pre-mix radiation quenching powders,** consistent with ingredients listed below:

Complete Vitamin/Mineral Fortification - ½ teaspoon powdered multi vitamin/mineral supplement, or simply open up one capsule of a complete multi-vitamin/mineral supplement into smoothie liquid. The complete vitamin portion (vitamins A through E) will offer broad-spectrum **antioxidant** protection, while the complete mineral portion (i.e., Ca/Mag/K/Sr), will help block 137Cs and 90Sr absorption (plus may offer superior radionuclide **elimination).**[826] Other critical minerals included are known to activate **Nrf2 antioxidant enzymes** (i.e., minerals copper, manganese, selenium, sulfur and zinc).

High Protein Immune Enhancement - 1 scoop high-grade whey containing immunoglobulins, enriched with Acetyl-L-Carnitine (ALCAR), plus beta-alanine (to boost internal carnosine levels), plus chondroitin sulfate - featuring sulfonation, **immunostimulation, vitagene, PGC-1 alpha, Nrf2 and connective tissue fortification**; or if allergic to high-grade whey, a suitable substitute would be 1 scoop select high-protein, gluten-free, delicious fermented whole grain-sprout powder.[827, 828, 829]

High Fiber/Probiotics - 1 heaping tablespoon of organic soluble and insoluble fibers including Chia seed powder (for fiber and omega 3 oils) - **antioxidant,**[830] plus 1 tablespoon organic pectin and 1 capsule probiotic emptied into smoothie liquid for radionuclide **elimination**.

To Make Cold: ¼ cup ice cubes made from filtered water.

Fruit and Vegetable Powder - Add in one scoop of super quenching fruit/vege/algae powder blend with an extra ¼ cup of filtered ice cubes (**super antioxidants+Nrf2** fortifying).

Natural Preservative to Retain Smoothie Freshness - 1/8th teaspoon buffered Vitamin C - **antioxidant.**

Malt and Texture Thickening - Add in 1 tablespoon barley malt syrup or rice malt syrup with a whole banana, pineapple, mangos, papaya, blueberries, grapes or other organic fruit of choice (adds in phytates and pectin for radionuclide **elimination**).

Other Flavorings - Ad lib allowable sweeteners and flavorings (i.e., vanilla, chocolate, fresh mint, cardamom/anise/licorice/cinnamon, etc…) of choice.

Recommended amounts to be ingested:

- 10-12 oz. smoothie for adults weighing over 150lbs once or more daily
- 8 oz smoothie for those weighing 100lbs to 149lbs once or more daily
- 6 oz smoothie for those weighing 50lbs to 99lbs once or more daily
- 4 oz smoothie or less for those under 50lbs once or more daily

Best Breakfast Smoothie – BB Smoothie (makes approximately 3 cups – 24 oz.):*

Preferred Liquids - 1 cup freshly squeezed organic orange juice (or other organic fruit juice of choice), featuring **antioxidants;** blended together with **specially formulated pre-mix radiation quenching powders,** or use the items below:

Complete Vitamin/Mineral Fortification - ½ teaspoon powdered multi vitamin/mineral supplement, or simply open up one capsule of a complete multi-vitamin/mineral supplement into smoothie liquid. The complete vitamin portion (Vitamins A through E) will offer broad-spectrum **antioxidant** protection, while the complete mineral portion (i.e., Ca/Mag/K/Sr), will help block 137Cs and 90Sr absorption (plus may offer superior radionuclide **elimination).**[831] Other critical minerals included are known to activate **Nrf2 antioxidant enzymes** (i.e., minerals copper, manganese, selenium, sulfur and zinc).

High Protein Immune Enhancement - 1 scoop high-grade whey containing immunoglobulins, enriched with Acetyl-L-Carnitine (ALCAR), plus beta-alanine (to boost internal Carnosine levels), plus chondroitin sulfate - featuring sulfonation, **immunostimulation, vitagene, PGC-1 alpha, Nrf2 and connective tissue fortification**; or if allergic to high-grade whey, a suitable substitute would be 1 scoop select high-protein, gluten-free, delicious fermented whole grain-sprout powder.[832, 833, 834]

High Fiber/Probiotics - 1 heaping tablespoon of organic soluble and insoluble fibers including Chia seed powder (for fiber and omega 3 oils) - **antioxidant,**[835] plus 1 tablespoon organic pectin and 1 capsule probiotic emptied into smoothie liquid for radionuclide **elimination**.

To Make Cold: ¼ cup ice cubes made from filtered water.

Fruit and Vegetable Powder - Add in one scoop of super quenching fruit/vege/algae powder blend with an extra ¼ cup of filtered ice cubes (**super antioxidants** + **Nrf2** fortifying).

Natural Preservative to Retain Smoothie Freshness - 1/8th teaspoon buffered Vitamin C - **antioxidant.**

Malt and Texture Thickening - Add in 1 tablespoon barley malt syrup or rice malt syrup with a whole banana, pineapple, mangos, papaya, blueberries, grapes or other organic fruit of choice (adds in phytates and pectin for radionuclide **elimination**).

Other Flavorings - Ad lib allowable sweeteners and flavorings (i.e., vanilla, chocolate, fresh mint, cardamom/anise/licorice/cinnamon, etc.) of choice.

Recommended amounts to be ingested:

- 10-12 oz. smoothie for adults weighing over 150lbs once or more daily
- 8 oz smoothie for those weighing 100lbs to 149lbs once or more daily
- 6 oz smoothie for those weighing 50lbs to 99lbs once or more daily
- 4 oz smoothie or less for those under 50lbs once or more daily

The below can be used as either for breakfast or as an in between meal refreshing drink, one per day.

Chelation/Creation Smoothie – CC Smoothie **(makes approximately three cups – 24 oz.):***

No fruits or vegetable powders for the CC Smoothie, except for bananas. Choice of:[836, 837]

Select and Specific Liquids - 1 cup It's Better Than Milk® (powdered tofu), organic soy milk (both rich in isoflavones, dipicolinic acid), *whole grain* rice milk or *whole grain* oat milk (both rich in Vit. B Complex, Vit. E Complex, tocotrienols and phytates from their bran and germ), featuring **antioxidants and radionuclide elimination;**[838] blended together with **specially formulated pre-mix radiation quenching powders,** or use the items below:

High Protein Immune Enhancement - 2 scoops high-grade whey enriched with Acetyl-L-Carnitine (ALCAR), plus beta-alanine, plus NAC, plus glucosamine sulfate - featuring **cysteine chelation, chitin chelation, immunostimulation, vitagene, PGC-1 alpha, Nrf2 and connective tissue** fortification; or if allergic to high-grade whey, a suitable substitute would be 1 scoop select high-protein, gluten-free, delicious fermented whole grain-sprout powder.

To Make Cold: ½ cup ice cubes made with filtered water.

Super Chelators - 2 tablespoons organic pectin- radionuclide **elimination** ½ teaspoon potassium/calcium alginate , plus 2 level teaspoons calcium bentonite clay, plus 1 capsule inositol hexaphosphate (IP-6, a form of phytic acid) emptied into liquid, **plus** 1 gram Glucosamine sulfate, with 1 capsule probiotics emptied into smoothie liquid - featuring **antioxidant**, **anti-mutagenic**, **immunostimulation**, **chitin chelation,** radionuclide **eliminatio**n.

Special Advisory: Folks with asthma or allergies to shellfish (i.e., shrimp) should consult their holistic physician before consuming this product. Glucosamine sulfate infrequently may cause allergic reactions in those susceptible.

Natural Preservative to Retain Smoothie Freshness - 1/8th teaspoon buffered Vitamin C - **antioxidant.**

Other Flavorings - Ad lib allowable sweeteners and flavorings of choice.

Recommended amounts to be ingested:

- 10-12 oz. a day for adults weighing over 150lbs
- 8 oz a day for those weighing 100lbs to 149lbs
- 6 oz a day for those weighing 50lbs to 99lbs
- 4 oz a day or less for those under 50lbs

Other Meal Item Suggestions

Breakfast: Whole oatmeal (rich in fiber plus phytates), high fiber oat cereals, or organic high fiber cereals of choice with suitable milk substitute and/or whole grain toast with 100% fruit jams (rich in pectin and antioxidants) with coconut butter, high-end hemp butter or preferred nut butter, but no trans-fat margarines.

Lunch: Salad, hard cheeses, olives, tomatoes, broccoli sprouts, fresh cilantro with homemade dressing using Udo's DHA 3-6-9 oil, or cold pressed organic sesame seed oil with spices, fresh herbs and balsamic vinegar. Add in blackened North Atlantic fish if desired, or switch this into dinner menu.

Soups: Several times weekly at lunch or dinner - miso soup plus sea vegetables and lightly cooked root vegetables, with or without Atlantic seafood, with rice noodles or brown rice. Consuming miso soup regularly provides significantly more protection over time. Miso soup (properly cooked miso paste with uncontaminated sea vegetables and cabbage family members) is anti-mutagenic and a good chelator of toxic metals aiding elimination.[839, 840]

Dinner: Whole grain pasta with marinara sauce and garlic toast with whole grain bread, or home made pizza with hard cheeses (i.e., no mozzarella), nitrate-free cured meats or vegetarian style with black olives, mushrooms grown in cultivation that is contaminant-free (mushrooms are superior chelators of radionuclides likely due to their rich content of norbadione).[841, 842]

Deserts: Organic pre-soaked/washed raw fruits, home-made sorbet ice cream, applesauce (or other easy-to-make fruit sauce), or organic fruit leather after lunch or the evening meal is one way to add adequate levels of pectin into anyone's diet.

For further information regarding dietary planning, see: **http://doctorapsley.com/GettingStarted.aspx.**For additional information about resources and supplies, see RESOURCES at the end of this chapter.

Protocols*

As I have already emphasized, (a) all exposure to radiation is cumulative; and (b) there is no safe level of radiation exposure. Therefore, it makes sense to incorporate easy-to-perform long-term radioprotection for you and your family. Greater still is the overall beneficial effects that select nutritional radio-protectors will have on anyone's health. It is like a double bonus - by protecting yourself from insidious radionuclide exposure, you are also helping your body to check premature aging, to help maintain strong immunity, and to keep your medical bills down in general.

For folks who scored themselves above in the radiation risk survey, the following protocols were developed to lessen the risks proportional to the totals.

- ✓ **The Basic Radiation Quenching Protocol (BRQP)** was designed to help lessen risks associated with folks *scoring a total of 1 or less.*
- ✓ **The Advanced Radiation Quenching Protocol (ARQP)** was designed to help lessen risks associated with a *score of 2 to 3.*
- ✓ **The Optimum Radiation Quenching Protocol (ORQP)** was designed to help lessen the risk associated with *scores of 4 or higher.*

In addition, below I cover protocol information for pregnant women, those who have suffered from acute radiation poisoning, and those who have suffered from poisoning but who are no longer being affected.

Super Nourishment – Basic Radiation Quenching Protocol (BRQP)*

Average adults (weighing +150lbs): For the first month, at breakfast consuming a CC Smoothie as described above may offer outstanding benefits. With the smoothie, it may be highly desirable to take:

- ✓ 3 capsules Antarctic krill oil at breakfast
- ✓ Providing no allergy to shellfish or iodine is present - North Atlantic kelp plus 200mg Vitamin C gradually increasing up to 5 capsules. Slowly increase kelp according to the guidelines spelled out in Chapter 3.

Lunch *and* dinner suggestions as part of a multi-course meal:

- ✓ Aim for three servings per week - miso soup, with tofu or suggested seafood, sea vegetables, cabbage family vegetables, daikon and brown rice.
- ✓ Bedtime:
- ✓ 3mg melatonin
- ✓ Also take 300mg of NAC
- ✓ And finally take 75mcg of selenium.

Young adults and larger children (weighing 100lbs - 149lbs): For the first month, at breakfast consuming a CC Smoothie as described above may offer outstanding benefits. With the smoothie, it may be highly desirable to take:

- ✓ 2 capsules Antarctic krill oil at breakfast
- ✓ Providing no allergy to shellfish or iodine is present - North Atlantic kelp plus 200mg Vitamin C gradually increasing up to 3 capsules. Slowly increase kelp according to the guidelines spelled out in Chapter 3.

Lunch *and* dinner suggestions as part of a multi-course meal:

- ✓ Aim for three servings per week - miso soup, with tofu or suggested seafood, sea vegetables, cabbage family vegetables, daikon and brown rice.

Bedtime:

- ✓ 3mg melatonin (chewable)
- ✓ Also take 300mg NAC
- ✓ And finally take 75mcg selenium.

For smaller children (weighing 50lbs - 99lbs): For the first month, at breakfast consuming a CC Smoothie as described above may offer outstanding benefits. With the smoothie, it may be highly desirable to take:

- ✓ 1 capsule Antarctic krill oil at breakfast (may be squished/pinched into smoothie)
- ✓ Providing no allergy to shellfish or iodine is present - North Atlantic kelp plus 200mg Vitamin C - 1 per meal.

Lunch *and* dinner suggestions as part of a multi-course meal:

- ✓ Aim for three servings per week - miso soup, with tofu or suggested seafood, sea vegetables, cabbage family vegetables, daikon and brown rice.

Bedtime:

- ✓ 2mg melatonin (chewable)
- ✓ Also take 100mg NAC
- ✓ And finally take 50mcg selenium.

For the very young (weighing less than 50lbs): For the first month, at breakfast consuming a CC Smoothie as described above may offer outstanding benefits. With the smoothie, it may be highly desirable to take:

- ✓ 1 capsule Antarctic krill oil at breakfast (may be squished/pinched into smoothie)
- ✓ Providing no allergy to shellfish or iodine is present - North Atlantic kelp plus 200mg Vitamin C - 1 per day mixed into smoothie, or juice or sweet potato or applesauce, etc...

Lunch *and* dinner suggestions as part of a multi-course meal:

- ✓ Aim for three servings per week - miso soup, with tofu or suggested seafood, sea vegetables, cabbage family vegetables, daikon and brown rice.

Bedtime:

- ✓ 500mcg (0.5mg) melatonin (chewable)
- ✓ Also take 25mg NAC
- ✓ And finally take 12.5mcg selenium.
- ✓ Contraindications to consuming any item above would include known food allergies or suspected intolerances.

Super Nourishment – Advanced Radiation Quenching Protocol (ARQP)*

Average adults (weighing +150lbs): For the first month, at breakfast consuming a CC Smoothie as described above may offer tremendous benefits. With the smoothie, it may be highly fortuitous to take:

- ✓ 3 capsules Antarctic krill oil at breakfast
- ✓ Up to 400iu natural Vitamin E with tocotrienols
- ✓ Providing no allergy to shellfish or iodine is present - North Atlantic kelp plus 200mg Vitamin C gradually increasing up to 5 capsules. Slowly increase kelp according to the guidelines spelled out in Chapter 3.

Lunch *and* dinner suggestions as part of a multi-course meal:

- ✓ Aim for three servings per week - miso soup, with tofu or suggested seafood, sea vegetables, cabbage family vegetables, daikon and brown rice
- ✓ 1 heaping scoop or 4 tablets of fruit/vegetable/herbal **antioxidant/Nrf2 factors**
- ✓ North Atlantic kelp plus 200mg Vitamin C, gradually increasing up to 5 capsules per meal.

Bedtime:

- ✓ 6mg melatonin
- ✓ Also take 300mg of NAC
- ✓ And finally take 150mcg of selenium.

Young adults and larger children (weighing 100lbs - 149lbs): For the first month, at breakfast consuming a CC Smoothie as described above may offer tremendous benefits. With the smoothie, it may be highly fortuitous to take:

- ✓ 2 capsules Antarctic krill oil at breakfast
- ✓ Up to 400iu natural Vitamin E with tocotrienols
- ✓ Providing no allergy to shellfish or iodine is present - North Atlantic kelp plus 200mg Vitamin C gradually increasing up to 3 capsules. Slowly increase kelp according to the guidelines spelled out in Chapter 3.

Lunch *and* dinner suggestions as part of a multi-course meal:

- ✓ Aim for three servings per week - miso soup, with tofu or suggested seafood, sea vegetables, cabbage family vegetables, daikon and brown rice
- ✓ 1 level scoop or 3 tablets of fruit/vegetable/herbal **antioxidant/Nrf2 factors**
- ✓ North Atlantic kelp plus 200mg Vitamin C, gradually increasing up to 3 capsules per meal.

Bedtime:

- ✓ 3mg melatonin
- ✓ Also take 150mg of NAC
- ✓ And finally take 75mcg of selenium.

For smaller children (weighing 50lbs - 99lbs): For the first month, at breakfast consuming a CC Smoothie as described above may offer tremendous benefits. With the smoothie, it may be highly fortuitous to take:

- ✓ 1 capsule Antarctic krill oil at breakfast (may be squished/pinched into smoothie)

- ✓ Up to 200iu natural Vitamin E with tocotrienols
- ✓ Providing no allergy to shellfish or iodine is present - North Atlantic kelp plus 200mg Vitamin C - 1 per meal.

Lunch *and* dinner suggestions as part of a multi-course meal:

- ✓ Aim for three servings per week - miso soup, with tofu or suggested seafood, sea vegetables, cabbage family vegetables, daikon and brown rice
- ✓ ½ scoop or 1 tablet of fruit/vegetable/herbal **antioxidant/Nrf2 factors**
- ✓ North Atlantic kelp plus 200mg Vitamin C - 1 per meal.

Bedtime:

- ✓ 1mg melatonin (chewable)
- ✓ Also take 50mg NAC
- ✓ And finally take 25mcg selenium.

For the very young (weighing less than 50lbs): For the first month, at breakfast consuming a CC Smoothie as described above may offer tremendous benefits. With the smoothie, it may be highly fortuitous to take:

- ✓ 1 capsule Antarctic krill oil at breakfast (may be squished/pinched into smoothie)
- ✓ Up to 50iu natural Vitamin E with tocotrienols
- ✓ Providing no allergy to shellfish or iodine is present - North Atlantic kelp plus 200mg Vitamin C - 1 per day mixed into smoothie, or juice or sweet potato or applesauce, etc...

Lunch *and* dinner suggestions as part of a multi-course meal:

- ✓ Aim for three servings per week - miso soup, with tofu or suggested seafood, sea vegetables, cabbage family vegetables, daikon and brown rice
- ✓ ½ scoop of fruit/vegetable/herbal **antioxidant/Nrf2 factors**.

Bedtime:

- ✓ 500mcg (0.5mg) melatonin (chewable)
- ✓ Also take 25mg NAC
- ✓ And finally take 12.5mcg selenium.

Contraindications to consuming any item above would include known food allergies or suspected intolerances.

Super Nourishment – Optimum Radiation Quenching Protocol (ORQP)*

Average adults (weighing +150lbs): For the first month, at breakfast consuming a CC Smoothie as described above may provide superior benefits. With the smoothie, it may be greatly rewarding to take:

- ✓ 3 capsules Antarctic krill oil at breakfast
- ✓ Up to 800iu natural Vitamin E with tocotrienols
- ✓ Up to 200mg CoQ10(H)
- ✓ Providing no allergy to shellfish or iodine is present - North Atlantic kelp plus 200mg Vitamin C gradually increasing up to 5 capsules. Slowly increase kelp according to the guidelines spelled out in Chapter 3.

Lunch *and* dinner suggestions as part of a multi-course meal:

- ✓ Aim for three servings per week - miso soup, with tofu or suggested seafood, sea vegetables, cabbage family vegetables, daikon and brown rice
- ✓ 1 heaping scoop or 4 tablets of fruit/vegetable/herbal **antioxidant/Nrf2 factors**
- ✓ North Atlantic kelp plus 200mg Vitamin C, gradually increasing up to 5 capsules per meal.

Bedtime:

- ✓ 10mg melatonin
- ✓ Also take 500mg of NAC
- ✓ And finally take 250mcg of selenium.

Young adults and larger children (weighing 100lbs - 149lbs): For the first month, at breakfast consuming a CC Smoothie as described above may provide superior benefits. With the smoothie, it may be greatly rewarding to take:

- ✓ 2 capsules Antarctic krill oil at breakfast
- ✓ Up to 100mg CoQ10(H)
- ✓ Up to 400iu natural Vitamin E with tocotrienols
- ✓ Providing no allergy to shellfish or iodine is present - North Atlantic kelp plus 200mg Vitamin C gradually increasing up to 3 capsules. Slowly increase kelp according to the guidelines spelled out in Chapter 3.

Lunch _and_ dinner suggestions as part of a multi-course meal:

- ✓ Aim for three servings per week - miso soup, with tofu or suggested seafood, sea vegetables, cabbage family vegetables, daikon and brown rice
- ✓ 1 level scoop or 3 tablets of fruit/vegetable/herbal **antioxidant/Nrf2 factors**
- ✓ North Atlantic kelp plus 200mg Vitamin C, gradually increasing up to 3 capsules per meal.

Bedtime:

- ✓ 6mg melatonin
- ✓ Also take 300mg of NAC
- ✓ And finally take 150mcg of selenium.

For smaller children (weighing 50lbs - 99lbs): For the first month, at breakfast consuming a CC Smoothie as described above may provide superior benefits. With the smoothie, it may be greatly rewarding to take:

- ✓ 1 capsule Antarctic krill oil at breakfast (may be squished/pinched into smoothie)
- ✓ Up to 50mg CoQ10(H)
- ✓ Up to 200iu natural Vitamin E with tocotrienols
- ✓ Providing no allergy to shellfish or iodine is present - North Atlantic kelp plus 200mg Vitamin C - 1 per meal.

Lunch *and* dinner suggestions as part of a multi-course meal:

- ✓ Aim for three servings per week - miso soup, with tofu or suggested seafood, sea vegetables, cabbage family vegetables, daikon and brown rice
- ✓ ½ scoop or 1 tablet of fruit/vegetable/herbal **antioxidant/Nrf2 factors**
- ✓ North Atlantic kelp plus 200mg Vitamin C - 1 per meal.

Bedtime:

- ✓ 3mg melatonin
- ✓ Also take 150mg of NAC
- ✓ And finally take 75mcg of selenium.

For the very young (weighing less than 50lbs): For the first month, at breakfast consuming a CC Smoothie as described above may provide superior benefits. With the smoothie, it may be greatly rewarding to take:

- ✓ 1 capsule Antarctic krill oil at breakfast (may be squished/pinched into smoothie)
- ✓ Up to 50iu natural Vitamin E with tocotrienols
- ✓ Providing no allergy to shellfish or iodine is present - North Atlantic kelp plus 200mg Vitamin C - 1 per day mixed into smoothie, or juice or sweet potato or applesauce, etc...

Lunch *and* dinner suggestions as part of a multi-course meal:

- ✓ Aim for three servings per week - miso soup, with tofu or suggested seafood, sea vegetables, cabbage family vegetables, daikon and brown rice
- ✓ ½ scoop of fruit/vegetable/herbal **antioxidant/Nrf2 factors**.

Bedtime:

- ✓ 500mcg (0.5mg) melatonin (chewable)
- ✓ Also take 25mg NAC
- ✓ And finally take 12.5mcg selenium.

Contraindications to consuming any item above would include known food allergies or suspected intolerances.

Additional Protocol Questions and Answers*

Q: If I am pregnant or am a nursing mother, what can I do to antidote my radiation exposure without harming my baby?

Answer. This is a great subject. If you have good reason to believe you are being exposed to traces of nuclear fall-out, going very slowly but "preemptively" is the key. Always proceed according to your holistic doctor's instructions. Never take baking soda if pregnant or nursing, unless instructed to do so by your physician. The below presumes you are already taking a HIGH POTENCY doctor approved prenatal or nursing multivitamin/multi-mineral supplement. Drink lots of purified water and eat lots of fiber!!! And do not use microwave ovens please!

It is always best to go slow and easy, while performing self-checks when incorporating nutritional supplements in pregnant or nursing mothers. For this reason, proceeding incrementally, with easy steps that build upon one another is the secret to success. This step-by-step procedure also allows time for the mother and young one to gently experience super nutrients over time. The step-by-step procedure also enables a fall-back position if required. For example, if say Step 2 causes no distress, but Step 3 brings some minor difficulties (i.e., such as mild nausea or headache), then it becomes clear to simply return to Step 2. After 3 days, it should become possible to once again resume slow incremental steps until the ideal protocol is attainable.

Contraindications to consuming any item below would include known food allergies or suspected intolerances.

Starting Schedule for Pregnant and Nursing Mothers: The first step is simply to take one AA Smoothie daily according to body weight.

If after three days of taking the above, no nausea or other discomfort arises if you are pregnant, or no mild skin rash or colic arises in your nursing baby, or any other suspicious symptom, continue on to the next schedule. If you experience difficulties of any kind, go through a process of elimination to find the offending item(s). Then restart the sequence.

Second Schedule for Pregnant and Nursing Mothers: The second step is simply to take one AA Smoothie daily according to body weight plus with the smoothie take:

- ✓ 1 capsule Antarctic krill oil at breakfast

- ✓ Providing no allergy to shellfish or iodine is present - North Atlantic kelp plus 200mg Vitamin C - 1 capsule.

Lunch *and* dinner suggestions as part of a multi-course meal: Aim for three servings per week - miso soup, with tofu or suggested seafood, sea vegetables, cabbage family vegetables, daikon and brown rice.

If after three days of taking above, no nausea or other discomfort arises if you are pregnant, or no mild skin rash or colic arises in your nursing baby, or any other suspicious symptom, continue on to the next schedule. If problems arise, discontinue until symptoms abate and resume the Starting Schedule.

Third Schedule for Pregnant and Nursing Mothers: The third step is simply to take one AA Smoothie daily according to body weight plus with the smoothie take:

- ✓ 2 capsules Antarctic krill oil at breakfast
- ✓ Providing no allergy to shellfish or iodine is present - North Atlantic kelp plus 200mg Vitamin C - 1 capsule.

Lunch *and* dinner suggestions as part of a multi-course meal:

- ✓ Aim for three servings per week - miso soup, with tofu or suggested seafood, sea vegetables, cabbage family vegetables, daikon and brown rice
- ✓ Providing no allergy to shellfish or iodine is present - North Atlantic kelp plus 200mg Vitamin C - 1 capsule per meal.

Bedtime:

- ✓ 1mg melatonin (chewable)

- ✓ Also take 50mg NAC
- ✓ And finally take 25mcg selenium.

If after three days of taking the above, no nausea or other discomfort arises if you are pregnant, or no mild skin rash or colic arises in your nursing baby, or any other suspicious symptom, continue onto the next schedule. If problems arise, discontinue until symptoms abate and resume the Second Schedule.

Fourth Schedule for Pregnant and Nursing Mothers: The fourth step is simply to take one AA Smoothie daily according to body weight plus with the smoothie take:

- ✓ 2 capsules Antarctic krill oil at breakfast
- ✓ Up to 400iu natural Vitamin E with tocotrienols
- ✓ Providing no allergy to shellfish or iodine is present - North Atlantic kelp plus 200mg Vitamin C - 2 capsules. Slowly increase kelp according to the guidelines spelled out in Chapter 3.

Lunch *and* dinner suggestions as part of a multi-course meal:

- ✓ Aim for three servings per week - miso soup, with tofu or suggested seafood, sea vegetables, cabbage family vegetables, daikon and brown rice
- ✓ ½ scoop or 1 tablet of fruit/vegetable/herbal **antioxidant/Nrf2 factors**
- ✓ North Atlantic kelp plus 200mg Vitamin C - 2 capsules per meal.

Bedtime:

- ✓ 1mg melatonin
- ✓ Also take 50mg of NAC
- ✓ And finally take 25mcg of selenium.

If after three days of taking the above, no nausea or other discomfort arises if you are pregnant, or no mild skin rash or colic arises in your nursing baby, or any other suspicious symptom, continue onto the next schedule. If problems arise, discontinue until symptoms abate and resume the Third Schedule.

Fifth Schedule for Pregnant and Nursing Mothers: The fifth step is simply to take one AA Smoothie daily according to body weight plus with the smoothie take:

- ✓ 2 capsules Antarctic krill oil at breakfast
- ✓ Up to 400iu natural Vitamin E with tocotrienols
- ✓ Providing no allergy to shellfish or iodine is present - North Atlantic kelp plus 200mg Vitamin C - 3 capsules. Slowly increase kelp according to the guidelines spelled out in Chapter 3.

Lunch *and* dinner suggestions as part of a multi-course meal:

- ✓ Aim for three servings per week - miso soup, with tofu or suggested seafood, sea vegetables, cabbage family vegetables, daikon and brown rice
- ✓ ½ scoop or 1 tablet of fruit/vegetable/herbal **antioxidant/Nrf2 factors**
- ✓ North Atlantic kelp plus 200mg Vitamin C - 3 capsules per meal.

Bedtime:

- ✓ 2mg melatonin
- ✓ Also take 100mg of NAC
- ✓ And finally take 50mcg of selenium.

If after three days of taking above, no nausea or other discomfort arises if you are pregnant, or no mild skin rash or colic arises in your nursing baby, or any other suspicious symptom, continue on to the next schedule. If problems arise, discontinue until symptoms abate and resume the Fourth Schedule.

Sixth Schedule for Pregnant and Nursing Mothers: The sixth step is simply to take one AA Smoothie daily according to body weight plus with the smoothie take:

- ✓ 2 capsules Antarctic krill oil at breakfast
- ✓ Up to 400iu natural Vitamin E with tocotrienols
- ✓ Providing no allergy to shellfish or iodine is present - North Atlantic kelp plus 200mg Vitamin C - 3 capsules. Slowly increase kelp according to the guidelines spelled out in Chapter 3.

Lunch *and* dinner suggestions as part of a multi-course meal:

- ✓ Aim for three servings per week - miso soup, with tofu or suggested seafood, sea vegetables, cabbage family vegetables, daikon and brown rice
- ✓ 1 level scoop or 3 tablets of fruit/vegetable/herbal **antioxidant/Nrf2 factors**
- ✓ North Atlantic kelp plus 200mg Vitamin C - 3 capsules per meal.

Bedtime:

- ✓ 2mg melatonin
- ✓ Also take 100mg of NAC
- ✓ And finally take 50mcg of selenium.

If after three days of taking above, no nausea or other discomfort arises if you are pregnant, or no mild skin rash or colic arises in your nursing baby, or any other suspicious symptom, continue onto the next schedule. If problems arise, discontinue until symptoms abate and resume the Fifth Schedule.

Seventh and Final Schedule for Pregnant and Nursing Mothers: The seventh step is simply to take one AA Smoothie daily according to body weight plus with the smoothie take:

- ✓ 2 capsules Antarctic krill oil at breakfast
- ✓ Up to 400iu natural Vitamin E with tocotrienols
- ✓ Up to 100mg CoQ10(H)
- ✓ Providing no allergy to shellfish or iodine is present - North Atlantic kelp plus 200mg Vitamin C - 3 capsules. Slowly increase kelp according to the guidelines spelled out in Chapter 3.

Lunch *and* dinner suggestions as part of a multi-course meal:

- ✓ Aim for three servings per week - miso soup, with tofu or suggested seafood, sea vegetables, cabbage family vegetables, daikon and brown rice
- ✓ 1 level scoop or 3 tablets of fruit/vegetable/herbal **antioxidant/Nrf2 factors**

- ✓ North Atlantic kelp plus 200mg Vitamin C - 3 capsules per meal.

Bedtime:

- ✓ 3mg melatonin
- ✓ Also take 150mg of NAC
- ✓ And finally take 75mcg of selenium.

If after three days of taking above, no nausea or other discomfort arises if you are pregnant, or no mild skin rash or colic arises in your nursing baby, or any other suspicious symptom, continue onto the next schedule. If problems arise, discontinue until symptoms abate and resume the Sixth Schedule.

The above schedules are designed to build intracellular glutathione stores via melatonin, selenium and NAC rapidly over time - the key molecule the body uses to eliminate radioactive metals through the bile - plus adequate antioxidant reserves such as Vitamin E which defend against lipid and genetic associated free-radicals.[843] The above list of nutrients also doubles as valuable nutritional items that all human beings can use, providing no allergy or sensitivity arises with their use.

Q: What can I do to antidote my Tissue Damage from radiation?

Answer: The AA, BB and CC Smoothie recipes above are designed to help stop ongoing damage from radiation poisoning, and then help eliminate the toxic particles from the body. After three to four months of use, it may be time to substitute a more regenerative smoothie program (see below).

Q: What if I am suffering from Acute Radiation Poisoning?

Answer: **Oral Acute Radiation Intervention Protocol (OARIP)** - For persons heavily exposed to radioactive particles, but still able to ingest foods and liquids, using the **OARIP** may be the best solution. The top medical priority is to permanently remove oneself from all possible future exposure.

Average adults (weighing +150lbs): Move away from all sources of radiation contamination. If exposed to fallout containing uranium and/or plutonium, for the first month, 30 minutes prior to eating or drinking anything, drink 1 pint purified water with 1 tablespoon baking soda mixed into water.[844] Later at breakfast, consuming a CC Smoothie as described above may be your most prudent course of action. With the smoothie, it may be essential to take:

- ✓ 6 capsules Antarctic krill oil at breakfast
- ✓ Up to 800iu natural Vitamin E with tocotrienols
- ✓ Up to 880mg CoQ10(H)
- ✓ 2,000mg gamma linolenic acid (GLA)
- ✓ 1,000mg NAC
- ✓ 40mg salicin from Willow Bark Complex[845]
- ✓ Providing no allergy to shellfish or iodine is present - North Atlantic kelp plus 200mg Vitamin C gradually increasing up to 5 capsules. Slowly increase kelp according to the guidelines spelled out in Chapter 3.

Lunch *and* dinner suggestions as part of a multi-course meal:

- ✓ Aim for three servings per week - miso soup, with tofu or suggested seafood, sea vegetables, cabbage family vegetables, daikon and brown rice
- ✓ 1 heaping scoop or 4 tablets of fruit/vegetable/herbal **antioxidant/Nrf2 factors**
- ✓ 1,000mg NAC
- ✓ 40mg salicin from Willow Bark Complex
- ✓ North Atlantic kelp plus 200mg Vitamin C, gradually increasing up to 5 capsules per meal.

Bedtime:

- ✓ 20mg melatonin
- ✓ 1,000mg NAC plus 500mcg organic selenium
- ✓ 40mg salicin from Willow Bark Complex.

Young adults and larger children (weighing 100lbs - 149lbs): For the first month, at breakfast consuming a CC Smoothie as described above may be your most prudent course of action. With the smoothie, it may be essential to take:

- ✓ 6 capsules Antarctic krill oil at breakfast
- ✓ Up to 440mg CoQ10(H)
- ✓ Up to 800iu natural Vitamin E with tocotrienols
- ✓ 500mg NAC
- ✓ 2,000mg gamma linolenic acid (GLA)
- ✓ 40mg salicin from Willow Bark Complex

- ✓ Providing no allergy to shellfish or iodine is present - North Atlantic kelp plus 200mg Vitamin C gradually increasing up to 3 capsules. Slowly increase kelp according to the guidelines spelled out in Chapter 3.

Lunch *and* dinner suggestions as part of a multi-course meal:

- ✓ Aim for three servings per week - miso soup, with tofu or suggested seafood, sea vegetables, cabbage family vegetables, daikon and brown rice
- ✓ 1 level scoop or 3 tablets of fruit/vegetable/herbal **antioxidant/Nrf2 factors**
- ✓ 500mg NAC
- ✓ 40mg salicin from willow bark complex
- ✓ North Atlantic kelp plus 200mg Vitamin C, gradually increasing up to 3 capsules per meal.

Bedtime:

- ✓ 10mg melatonin (chewable)
- ✓ 500mg NAC plus 250mcg organic selenium.

For smaller children (weighing 50lbs - 99lbs): For the first month, at breakfast consuming a CC Smoothie as described above may be your most prudent course of action. With the smoothie, it may be essential to take:

- ✓ 3 capsules Antarctic krill oil at breakfast (may be squished/pinched into smoothie)
- ✓ Up to 220mg CoQ10(H)
- ✓ Up to 400iu natural Vitamin E with tocotrienols
- ✓ 1,000mg gamma linolenic acid (GLA)

- ✓ 250mg NAC
- ✓ 40mg salicin from willow bark complex
- ✓ Providing no allergy to shellfish or iodine is present - North Atlantic kelp plus 200mg Vitamin C - 1 per meal.

Lunch *and* dinner suggestions as part of a multi-course meal:

- ✓ Aim for three servings per week - miso soup, with tofu or suggested seafood, sea vegetables, cabbage family vegetables, daikon and brown rice
- ✓ ½ scoop or 1 tablet of fruit/vegetable/herbal **antioxidant/Nrf2 factors**
- ✓ 250mg NAC
- ✓ North Atlantic kelp plus 200mg Vitamin C - 1 per meal.

Bedtime:

- ✓ 5mg melatonin (chewable)
- ✓ 250mg NAC plus 125mcg organic selenium
- ✓ 40mg salicin from willow bark complex.

For the very young (weighing less than 50lbs): For the first month, at breakfast consuming a CC Smoothie as described above may be your most prudent course of action. With the smoothie, it may be essential to take:

- ✓ 1 capsule Antarctic krill oil at breakfast (may be squished/pinched into smoothie)
- ✓ Up to 50iu natural Vitamin E with tocotrienols
- ✓ 250mg GLA squished/pinched into smoothie liquid
- ✓ 50mg NAC

- ✓ Providing no allergy to shellfish or iodine is present - North Atlantic kelp plus 200mg Vitamin C - 1 per day mixed into smoothie, or juice or sweet potato or applesauce, etc...

Lunch *and* dinner suggestions as part of a multi-course meal:

- ✓ Aim for three servings per week - miso soup, with tofu or suggested seafood, sea vegetables, cabbage family vegetables, daikon and brown rice
- ✓ ½ scoop of fruit/vegetable/herbal **antioxidant/Nrf2 factors**.
- ✓ 50mg NAC

Bedtime:

- ✓ 1mg melatonin (chewable)
- ✓ 50mg NAC plus 25mcg selenium.

Contraindications to consuming any item above would include known food allergies or suspected intolerances. Uranium and/or plutonium exposure: consider baking soda dosage schedule.

Use of Baking Soda

Under a doctor's supervision, baking soda (sodium bicarbonate or $NaHCO_3$) coupled to complete anti-inflammatory intervention plus the immediately above protocols are tools of choice to remove these toxic metals from the body quickly.

Baking soda should be taken only on *rare* occasions, that is, only if exposures to uranium or plutonium can be confirmed, even in trace amounts, for your area. Baking soda is an efficient means to remove metals quickly (especially uranium), and especially if used in combination with other antioxidants.[846, 847, 848]

There are several medical conditions including pregnancy which contradict taking *baking soda,* so be sure you have doctor's clearance before consuming *baking soda.* Taking baking soda once weekly should pose no health threat if no other medical conditions are present that require restriction of sodium intake. For adults with no medical contraindications, and who have good reason to believe they have been exposed to traces of radioactive fall-out, especially uranium, baking soda may be a tool for you and your doctor to consider. For those weighing over 150 pounds (70 kilograms), take 1 tablespoon of baking soda and mix into 1 pint water or juice. You doctor may suggest you take this solution once daily for seven days on an empty stomach.

For the more serious exposures, doctors may suggest adults ingest up to 7 teaspoons of baking soda daily in divided dosages on an empty stomach for short-term treatment. When taken over six consecutive days, significant decontamination may be achieved. But the route and rate of administration must be carefully considered by the physician. Another acceptable dosage schedule is to perform the above every other day for two weeks on, then resting for two weeks off of the baking soda schedule.

Parenteral Anti-Inflammation/ Antidote Protocol

In the extremely unlikely event of more grave situations, your physician may consider intravenous administration over 60 minutes of various mitigators to radiation poisoning. This section especially applies to those unable to ingest the super nutritional items in the above radiation quenching protocols. In addition to the conventional choice, among the finest complementary nutraceuticals are:

- ✓ 5% solution of baking soda (in D-5-W for a total of 500cc)
- ✓ Reduced glutathione (2gm)
- ✓ Reduced CoQ10 (300mg)
- ✓ Sodium ascorbate (10gm)
- ✓ Omega 3 oils (2gm)
- ✓ NAC (5gm) and
- ✓ Elemental selenium (1mg) as sodium selenite.

The above formula can be administered daily over the course of a week or two, with good success where the patient is incapable of ingesting oral supplements.

If skin exposure has been confirmed, then infrared saunas using niacin and intense sweats are key. Be sure to collect the sweat on towels during the twice daily 30 minute treatments, and then properly dispose of the towels.

For additional Regeneration Effect resources and professional-grade supplies at discounted prices, see: http://doctorapsley.com/EssentialLinks.aspx

The Regeneration Effect™ Protocol (REP)

Providing the current and future exposure to radiation has been eliminated, folks who feel they accrued tissue damage from radiation may also wish to consider a regeneration approach. In fact, anyone with tissue damage resulting from extended free-radical pathology (ex-smokers or sufferers of chronic degenerative illnesses), may wish to consider a regeneration approach to their current health status. My family and I also use this regeneration protocol as our long-term maintenance program.

The Regeneration Effect™ requires special "priming" to jump start sluggish or damaged repair systems of the body. In essence, we start priming the entire system from the cell level up. In this manner, it becomes consistently possible to accelerate repair and/or bring about unscheduled repair that would not ordinarily occur.

Pillar 1: Detoxification

The priming phase works hand in hand with detoxification. Detoxification is the First Pillar of The Regeneration Effect™. The REP contains many of the same ingredients that help eliminate any remaining toxic metal particles, including those which are radioactive, from the body. Detoxification starts and continues with (a) a high fiber diet rich in pectin and alginate, as well as phytates. Additionally, (b) consuming large amounts of special water is important over the long run. Both are found in raw juices and raw foods (i.e., salads). Some folks also like to invest in special water filtration systems that concentrate alkaline minerals in the water. For further information on such a diet, see RESOURCES at the end of this chapter.

The main ingredients of the priming phase are three fold: (a) select raw proteins from highest quality whey, grain-sprout concentrate and/or algae, (b) colloidal minerals from organic raw foods, and (c) pure alkaline water from raw foods. For ease and simplicity, you can accomplish the entire priming phase with the regular consumption of the previously described regenerative smoothies by combining them with freshly juiced fruits and vegetables.

These three items along with proper detoxification provide cells the very best materials possible for achieving optimal function.

Pillar 2: Maximal Oxygenation (MaxO$_2$)

As previously mentioned in Chapter 6, restoring optimal numbers and function of cellular mitochondria via PGC-1α enables best use of oxygen at the cell level. In addition to stimulating higher levels of PGC-1α, plentiful supplies of chlorophyll greatly add to the body's ability to transport oxygen throughout the tissues. Finally, CoQ10(H) excites the final steps of aerobic (oxygen required) energy production in every cell of the body, plus protects heart function.

Regular exercise in fresh air, such as physical yoga, swimming, walking, exercising with oxygen or breathing in oxygen while in a sauna are all excellent ways to optimize cellular oxygenation. Also, The next step is to induce accelerated and/or unscheduled repair with select foods that Super-Nourishment - Pillar Three.

Pillar 3: Super Nourishment

Radiation toxicity from any source (including the after effects of radioablative therapy in cancer treatment), may be reversed by the use of colloidal Regeneration Factors or **cRFs**™.[849, 850, 851, 852]

cRFs™ also derive from select raw foods that contain high amounts of RNA or nucleoproteins as found in food-grade algae, organ meats, nuts and seeds, sprouts and bee pollen (which are microscopic seeds).

Folks with a history of gout cannot take high amounts of these select foods, but usually can handle some intake providing the source is *raw*. Excellent sources of raw RNA are low-temperature dried algae and freeze-dried glandular capsules. Folks with a history of gout must also consider optimum consumption of pure water as a part of the regular daily schedule.

Pillar 4: BioEnergetics

We repair at certain rates of speed at specific times of the day by way of our intrinsic circadian rhythm. For example, cell and tissue repair becomes greatly facilitated when we enter deep slow wave sleep (or SWS) and REM sleep periods.[853,854,855] Specifically, our circadian rhythm determines the extent and timing of cell repair by turning on and off both apoptosis and autophagy, as well as immune related repair.[856]

The REP supports this fourth pillar of regeneration by including herbs and nutrients that stimulate both apoptosis as well as autophagy. This was covered in previous chapters. But the REP's most influential nutrient in this regard would appear to be melatonin.[857] For example, a most crippling long-term effect of ionizing radiation is that it breaks apart our DNA. Our intrinsic circadian rhythm controls the DNA repair process[858] and melatonin redoubles the efforts of the circadian rhythm to do so.[859] Just as importantly, melatonin facilitates our immune response, the spearhead to regenerative repair.[860,861]

Also, the REP supports PGC-1α stimulation to induce genesis of essential cellular mitochondria by way of select amino acids, resveratrol and lipoic acid as covered in previous chapters.

Interestingly, there appears to be a timing factor to DNA repair verses the genesis of mitochondria. For example, the excitation of DNA repair by melatonin may be interfered with by nutrients used to excite mitochondrial production. Timing is the key. Specifically, resveratrol increases PGC-1α levels by way of another chemical called SIRT-1. Yet, too much SIRT-1 stymies both DNA repair and apoptosis.[862] To avoid such a time-sensitive conflict, melatonin is only to be taken at bedtime (night time), while the PGC-1α nutrients are only to be taken during daytime (light time) hours. In this manner, restful regenerative sleep is more easily attained.

Adequate restful sleep is essential for everyone who is on a regeneration program.[863, 864] For those with serious illness (especially in chronic inflammatory states), no less than 10 hours deep sleep is suggested daily.[865, 866, 867]

Another excellent and relaxing energetic method that appears to amplify regeneration is music and sound therapy, or Bioacoustics.[868, 869, 870, 871, 872] Also, tapping on select acupuncture points along the face and hands while mentally reciting positive affirmations for about 10 minutes twice daily is also a great way to support and amplify the healing process.[873]

Throughout the ages, prayer, meditation and fasting (via autophagy) are also tried and true methods to activate the Fourth Pillar of The Regeneration Effect™.[874, 875]

Regeneration Effect Protocol

Average adults (weighing +150lbs): For the first month, at breakfast use a CC Smoothie as described above. Thereafter, use the AA and/or BB Smoothie recipes ad lib. With the breakfast smoothie take:

- ✓ 3 capsules Antarctic krill oil at breakfast (rich in essential phospholipids such as PS and PC)[876]
- ✓ Up to 800iu natural Vitamin E with tocotrienols
- ✓ Up to 220mg CoQ10(H)
- ✓ Up to 100mg R-alpha lipoic acid (R-ALA)
- ✓ Up to 600mg arginine *alpha*-ketoglutarate complex or up to 1 gram beta-alanine
- ✓ Up to 100mg resveratrol complex
- ✓ 2 capsules cold sterilized immune glandular supplement containing uncontaminated sources of freeze-dried thymus, spleen and bone marrow
- ✓ Providing no allergy to shellfish or iodine is present - North Atlantic kelp plus 200mg Vitamin C gradually increasing up to 5 capsules. Slowly increase kelp according to the guidelines spelled out in Chapter 3.

Lunch <u>*and*</u> dinner suggestions as part of a multi-course meal:

- ✓ Aim for three servings per week - miso soup, with tofu or suggested seafood, sea vegetables, cabbage family vegetables, daikon and brown rice
- ✓ 1 heaping scoop or 4 tablets of fruit/vegetable/herbal **antioxidant/Nrf2 factors**
- ✓ Up to 600mg arginine *alpha*-ketoglutarate complex or up to 1 gram beta-alanine
- ✓ Up to 100mg resveratrol complex

- ✓ 2 capsules immune glandular supplement containing uncontaminated sources of freeze-dried thymus, spleen and bone marrow
- ✓ North Atlantic kelp plus 200mg Vitamin C, gradually increasing up to 5 capsules per meal.

Bedtime:

- ✓ 20mg melatonin
- ✓ 1,000mg NAC plus 500mcg organic selenium.

Overdoing selenium is possible. The first sign of taking too much selenium is acceleated hair loss, which is 100% reversible by simply discontinuing selenium.

Young adults and larger children (weighing 100lbs - 149lbs): For the first month, at breakfast use a BB Smoothie or CC Smoothie as described above. With the smoothie take:

- ✓ 3 capsules Antarctic krill oil at breakfast
- ✓ Up to 100mg CoQ10(H)
- ✓ Up to 800iu natural Vitamin E with tocotrienols
- ✓ Up to 100mg R-alpha lipoic acid (R-ALA)
- ✓ Up to 300mg arginine *alpha*-ketoglutarate complex or 1 gram beta-alanine
- ✓ Up to 100mg resveratrol complex
- ✓ 1 capsule Immune glandular supplement containing uncontaminated sources of freeze-dried thymus, spleen and bone marrow

- ✓ Providing no allergy to shellfish or iodine is present - North Atlantic kelp plus 200mg Vitamin C gradually increasing up to 3 capsules. Slowly increase kelp according to the guidelines spelled out in Chapter 3.

Lunch *and* dinner suggestions as part of a multi-course meal:

- ✓ Aim for three servings per week - miso soup, with tofu or suggested seafood, sea vegetables, cabbage family vegetables, daikon and brown rice.
- ✓ 1 level scoop or 3 tablets of fruit/vegetable/herbal **antioxidant/Nrf2 factors**
- ✓ Up to 300mg arginine *alpha*-ketoglutarate complex or 1 gram beta-alanine
- ✓ Up to 100mg Resveratrol Complex
- ✓ 1 capsule immune glandular supplement containing uncontaminated sources of freeze-dried thymus, spleen and bone marrow
- ✓ North Atlantic kelp plus 200mg Vitamin C, gradually increasing up to 3 capsules per meal.

Bedtime:

- ✓ 10mg melatonin (chewable)
- ✓ 500mg NAC plus 250mcg organic selenium.

For smaller children (weighing 50lbs - 99lbs): For the first month, at breakfast use a BB Smoothie or CC Smoothie as described above. With the smoothie take:

- ✓ 1 capsule Antarctic krill oil at breakfast (may be squished/pinched into smoothie)

- ✓ Up to 50mg CoQ10(H)
- ✓ Up to 200iu natural Vitamin E with tocotrienols
- ✓ Providing no allergy to shellfish or iodine is present - North Atlantic kelp plus 200mg Vitamin C - 1 per meal.
- ✓ Lunch _and_ dinner suggestions as part of a multi-course meal:
- ✓ Aim for three servings per week - miso soup, with tofu or suggested seafood, sea vegetables, cabbage family vegetables, daikon and brown rice
- ✓ ½ scoop or 1 tablet of fruit/vegetable/herbal **antioxidant/Nrf2 factors**
- ✓ 1 capsule immune glandular supplement containing uncontaminated sources of freeze-dried thymus, spleen and bone marrow
- ✓ North Atlantic kelp plus 200mg Vitamin C - 1 per meal.

Bedtime:

- ✓ 1mg melatonin (chewable)
- ✓ 50mg NAC plus 25mcg organic selenium.

For the very young (weighing less than 50lbs): For the first month, at breakfast use a BB Smoothie or CC Smoothie as described above. With the smoothie take:

- ✓ 1 capsule Antarctic krill oil at breakfast (may be squished/pinched into smoothie)
- ✓ Up to 50iu natural Vitamin E with tocotrienols

- ✓ ½ capsule immune glandular supplement containing uncontaminated sources of freeze-dried thymus, spleen and bone marrow emptied into smoothie liquid
- ✓ Providing no allergy to shellfish or iodine is present - North Atlantic kelp plus 200mg Vitamin C - 1 per day mixed into smoothie, or juice or sweet potato or applesauce, etc...

Lunch *and* dinner suggestions as part of a multi-course meal:

- ✓ Aim for three servings per week - miso soup, with tofu or suggested seafood, sea vegetables, cabbage family vegetables, daikon and brown rice
- ✓ ½ scoop of fruit/vegetable/herbal **antioxidant/Nrf2 factors**.

Bedtime:

- ✓ 500mcg (0.5mg) melatonin (chewable)
- ✓ Also take 25mg NAC
- ✓ And finally take 12.5mcg selenium.

Contraindications to consuming any item above would include known food allergies or suspected intolerances.

Resources

For further information on how to design, set up and implement diets consistent with the Four Pillars of The Regeneration Effect™, see: http://doctorapsley.com/GettingStarted.aspx.

For additional Regeneration Effect resources and professional-grade supplies, see:
http://doctorapsley.com/EssentialLinks.aspx.

Conclusion

As of September 30th, 2011, the Southern Hemisphere remains as our planet's least contaminated haven from radioactive fallout. Although radioactive fallout has penetrated below the equator, the levels are miniscule compared to those found in the Northern Hemisphere. Food sources from the Southern Hemisphere are critical to the survival of humankind, and must be protected from the threat of future contamination.

Unfortunately, the threat to the Southern Hemisphere could not currently be greater. Australia possesses 40% of the world's known reserves of uranium. Under the previous laws, the uranium was mined via tunnel networks, similar to many coal mining operations.

But recently, authority was given to multiple Australian mining companies to begin "above straight-down" mining which simply digs straight down into the earth with massive earth digging equipment.[877] The resulting dust storms from such a procedure will release vast tonnage of finely powdered radioactive uranium into the Southern Hemisphere's atmosphere and contaminate the only remaining region on earth relatively free from radioactive fallout.[878, 879]

This must be stopped now because time is running out. There is an excellent short video you can watch to first understand what is looming on the horizon, and who to contact to help stop this travesty from happening down under. It is a concern we must all share, or we will surely all suffer the consequences.

For further information, see the following link and watch the video at: http://www.roxstop-action.org/#!__site

You can also now view a very complete documentary on the Fukushima aftermath at:
http://www.youtube.com/watch?v=LethPJ9Vd8Y.

May we all find the way to make this a better world for ourselves and our children. Good luck everyone, you'll need it.

Regeneration Effect
Highly Suggested Reading:

- ✓ *Hypothyroidism Type 2*, by Mark Starr, MD.
- ✓ *Healing is Voltage: The Key to Pain Control and Chronic Disease*, by Jerry Tennant, MD.
- ✓ Sound (BioAcoustics) Therapy - see: http://www.soundhealthoptions.com/pdf/JBAB_II.pdf
- ✓ *The Regeneration Effect*, Volume 1, Fully Revised, by John W. Apsley, MD(E), ND, DC (due out late 2011 or early 2012).
- ✓ *The Regeneration Effect: Curing (vs. Controlling) Terminal Cancer*, Volume 3, by John W. Apsley, MD(E), ND, DC (due out Spring/Summer 2012).

Endnotes

1 See: http://wisequotes.org/nuclear-power-is-one-hell-of-a-way-to-boil-water.

2 See: http://www.greenpeace.org/usa/en/campaigns/nuclear/.

3 See Lovins AB, Sheikh I. The Nuclear Illusion, A White Paper: http://www.rmi.org/rmi/Library/E08-01_NuclearIllusion.

4 Lovins AB, Sheikh I. Lovins and Sheikh defend their work in 'The Nuclear Illusion.' Grist: Nuclear Deterrence. 2008 Jun 19, 1:30 PM; see: http://www.grist.org/article/nuclear-deterrence.

5 Sokolski HD. Nuclear Power's Global Expansion: Weighing Its Costs and Risks [Kindle Edition]. File Size: 5452 KB, Amazon Digital Services, Language: English, ASIN: B0050P4S12. See: http://www.amazon.com/Nuclear-Powers-Global-Expansion-ebook/dp/B0050P4S12/ref=sr_1_17?ie=UTF8&qid=1314764393&sr=8-17

6 McKeating J. Nuclear power is in last place in the race against climate change. Greenpeace. 2011 Jul 22, 10:29; see: http://www.greenpeace.org/usa/en/news-and-blogs/campaign-blog/nuclear-power-is-in-last-place-in-the-race-ag/blog/35841/

7 See: http://www.greenpeace.org/usa/Global/usa/planet3 /publications/nukes/Decommissioning%20Risks.pdf

8 Buettner D. The blue zones: lessons for living longer from the people who've lived the longest. *National Geographic*. Washington, D.C., 2008.

9 Gould JM, Goldman BA. *Deadly Deceit: Low Level Radiation High Level Cover-Up*. Four Walls Eight Windows, NY, NY, 1990; pp. 95-109.

10 For example, cogeneration of gas coupled to steam turbine electrical generation improves electrical energy yield from 40%-60% to 90% (see: http://www.scribd.com/doc/15000531/Gas-Turbines-for-Electrical-Power-Production). Also, see supercritical heated water systems at: http://www.iaus.com/BladelessTurbine.aspx.

11 See: http://en.wikipedia.org/wiki/List_of_civilian_nuclear_accidents

12 Contrary to power company figures, cost of nuclear power generation highest: research. *The Mainichi Daily News*. Japan, 2011 Jul 23; see: http://mdn.mainichi.jp/features/archive/news/2011/07/20110723p2a00m0na011000c.html

13 See: http://news.businessweek.com/article.asp?documentKey=1376-LQ0I2N0YHQ0W01-4B2UHQGJDPRPMFG9AKUVDE7FR5

14 Gray L. Public to pay for new nuclear era. *The Telegraph*, Earth News. UK, 2010 Oct 19; see: http://www.telegraph.co.uk/earth/earthnews/8071311/Public-to-pay-for-new-nuclear-era.html

15 Obiko N, Bandel C. Atomic cleanup cost goes to Japan's taxpayers, may spur liability shift. *Bloomberg*. 2011 Mar 23;See: http://www.bloomberg.com/news/2011-03-23/nuclear-cleanup-cost-goes-to-japan-s-taxpayers-may-spur-liability-shift.html

16 The KiKK study – Kaatsch P, et al. Leukemia in young children living in the vicinity of German nuclear power plants. *Int J Cancer*. 2008; 1220:721-26.

17 Baker PJ, Hoel DG. Meta-analysis of standardized incidence and mortality rates of childhood leukemia in proximity to nuclear facilities. *Eur J Cancer Care*. 2007:16:355-63.

18 Laurier D, et al. Epidemiological studies of leukemia in children and young adults around nuclear facilities: a critical review. *Rad Prot Dosim*. 2008; 132:182-90.

19 Caldicott H. The medical and economic costs of nuclear power. Online Opinion. Australia, 2009 Sep 14; see: http://www.onlineopinion.com.au/view.asp?article=9422&page=0.

20 Jack, A., *Let Thy Food Be Thy Medicine*. One Peaceful World Press, Becket, MA, 1991, p. 87-9.

21 Schechter SR. *Fighting Radiation with Foods, Herbs & Vitamins*. East-West Health Books, Brookline, MA, p. 6, 85-6.

22 See: http://www.helencaldicott.com/2011/07/internal-radioactive-emitters-invisible-tasteless-and-odorless/.

23 Sun MF, et al. Search for novel remedies to augment radiation resistance of Inhabitants of Fukushima and Chernobyl disasters: identifying DNA repair protein XRCC4 inhibitors. *J Biomol Struct Dyn*. 2011 Oct;29(2):325-37.

24 See: http://www.krill-oil-benefits.com/phospholipids.php.

25 Ling GN. A new theoretical foundation for the polarized-oriented multilayer theory of cell water and for inanimate systems demonstrating long-range dynamic structuring of water molecules. *Physiol Chem Phys Med NMR*. 2003;35(2):91-130.

26 Yablokov AV, Nesterenko VB, Nesterenko AV. Chernobyl: Consequences of the catastrophe for people and the environment. *Ann N Y Acad Sci*. (paperback ed.) 2009 Dec;1181(1). Wiley-Blackwell.

27 Graeub R. *The Petkau Effect: Nuclear Radiation, People and Trees*. Four Walls Eight Windows, NY, 1992.

28 Fliedner TM, Graessle DH. Hematopoietic cell renewal systems: mechanisms of coping and failing after chronic exposure to ionizing radiation. *Radiat Environ Biophys*. 2008 Feb;47(1):63-9.

29 Graeub R. *The Petkau Effect: Nuclear Radiation, People and Trees*. Four Walls Eight Windows, NY, 1992.

30 Null G, et al. What physicians should know about the biological effects of ingested fission products. *Townsend Letter for Doctors & Patients*. 1993 Aug-/Sep;(121/122):812.

31 Vanderplog HA, et al. Bioaccumulation Factors for Radionuclides in Freshwater Biota. ORNL-5002 (1975), Environmental Sciences Division Publication, Number 783, Oak Ridge National Laboratory, Oak Ridge, TN.

32 Clark JU, McFarland VA. Assessing Bioaccumulation in Aquatic Organisms Exposed to Contaminated Sediments. Miscellaneous Paper D-91-2 (1991). Environmental Laboratory. Waterways Experiment Station, Vicksburg, MS.

33 Watson WS, et al. Radionuclides in seals and porpoises in the coastal waters around the *UK. Sci Total Environ*. 1999 Aug 30;234(1-3):1-13.

34 Fessenko SV, et al. An extended critical review of twenty years of countermeasures used in agriculture after the Chernobyl accident. *Sci Total Environ*. 2007 Sep 20;383(1-3):1-24.

35 Gong YF, et al. Suppression of radioactive strontium absorption by sodium alginate in animals and human subjects. *Biomed Environ Sci.* 1991 Sep;4(3):273-82.

36 Nesterenko VB, Nesterenko AV. Decorporation of Chernobyl radionuclides. *Ann N Y Acad Sci.* 2009 Nov;1181(1):303-10.

37 Robbins ME, Bourland JD, Cline JM, Wheeler KT, Deadwyler SA. A model for assessing cognitive impairment after fractionated whole-brain irradiation in nonhuman primates. *Radiat Res.* 2011 Apr;175(4):519-25.

38 García-Pérez A, Sierrasesumaga L, Narbona-García J, Calvo-Manuel F, Aguirre-Ventalló M. Neuropsychological evaluation of children with intracranial tumors: Impact of treatment modalities *Medical and Pediatric Oncology* 1994;23(2):116-23.

39 Patel SK, Mullins WA, O'Neil SH, Wilson K. Neuropsychological differences between survivors of supratentorial and infratentorial brain tumours. *J Intellect Disabil Res.* 2011 Jan;55(1):30-40.

40 Lowe XR, Bhattacharya S, Marchetti F, Wyrobek AJ. Early brain response to low-dose RADIATION exposure involves molecular networks and pathways associated with cognitive functions, advanced aging and Alzheimer's disease. *Radiat Res.* 2009 Jan;171(1):53-65.

41 Tian Y, Shi Z, Yang S, Chen Y, Bao S. Changes in myelin basic protein and demyelination in the rat brain within 3 months of single 2-, 10-, or 30-Gy whole-brain radiation treatments. *J Neurosurg.* 2008 Nov;109(5):881-8.

42 Akiyama K, Tanaka R, Sato M, Takeda N. Cognitive dysfunction and histological findings in adult rats one year after whole brain irradiation. *Neurol Med Chir (Tokyo).* 2001 Dec;41(12):590-8.

43 Rice D, Barone S Jr. Critical periods of vulnerability for the developing nervous system: evidence from humans and animal models. *Environ Health Perspect.* 2000 Jun;108 Suppl 3:511-33.

44 Wambi CO, et al. Protective effects of dietary antioxidants on proton total-body irradiation-mediated hematopoietic cell and animal survival. *Radiat Res*. 2009 Aug;172(2):175-86.

45 Abd-El-Fattah AA, El-Sawalhi MM, Rashed ER, El-Ghazaly MA. Possible role of vitamin E, coenzyme Q10 and rutin in protection against cerebral ischemia/reperfusion injury in irradiated rats. *Int J Radiat Biol.* 2010 Dec;86(12):1070-8.

46 Meng X, Riordan NH. Cancer is a functional repair tissue. Med Hypotheses. 2006;66(3):486-90.

47 Ling S, et al. An EGFR-ERK-SOX9 Signaling Cascade Links Urothelial Development and Regeneration to Cancer. *Cancer Res.* 2011 Jun 1;71(11):3812-21.

48 DuFort CC, Paszek MJ, Weaver VM. Balancing forces: architectural control of mechanotransduction. *Nat Rev Mol Cell Biol.* 2011 May;12(5):308-19.

49 Weber A, Boege YT, Reisinger F, Heikenwälder M. Chronic liver inflammation and hepatocellular carcinoma: persistence matters. *Swiss Med Wkly.* 2011 May 10;141:w13197.

50 Graeub R. *The Petkau Effect.* 2nd edition, Four Walls Eight Windows, New York, NY (1994).

51 Health Risks from Exposure to Low Levels of Ionizing Radiation: BEIR VII – Phase 2 Committee to Assess Health Risks from Exposure to Low Levels of Ionizing Radiation. National Research Council. For free download see: http://www.nap.edu/catalog/11340.html.

52 See: http://en.wikipedia.org/wiki/Nuclear_weapon.

53 See: http://www-ns.iaea.org/downloads/rw/waste-safety/north-test-site-final.pdf.

54 See page 318 at: http://www.iaea.org/inis/collection/NCLCollectionStore/_Public/31/017/31017713.pdf.

55 1 Becquerel (1 Bq) of Plutonium per Kilogram of foodstuff exceeds the permissible dose according to the Codex Alimentarius (C.A.). 1,000 Becquerels (1 X 103 Becquerels or 1 kBq) of Cesium per Kilogram of foodstuff exceeds the permissible dose according to C.A. The Chernobyl Catastrophe released – 12 Quadrillion 1 kBqs – of radiation.

56 See page 317 at: http://www.iaea.org/inis/collection/NCLCollectionStore/_Public/31/017/31017713.pdf.

57 Napier BA. Selection of Dominant Radionuclides for Phase I of the Hanford Environmental Dose Reconstruction Project, Appendices D & E. PNL-7231 HEDR, 1991 Jul. Also see: http://hanford-downwinders.tribe.net/thread/27ac20d9-46ee-4fd7-9fae-15a0be3a7665.

58 Hanson LA. Radioactive Waste Contamination of Soil and Groundwater at the Hanford Site. University of Idaho, *Principles of Environmental Toxicology* 2000 Nov; p. 4. See: http://www.agls.uidaho.edu/etox/resources/case_studies/HANFORD.PDF. [Ref: 437 million Curies = 16,169 X 10^{15} Bq total radioactivity]

59 Gould JA. *The Enemy Within: The High Cost of Living Near Nuclear Reactors.* Four Walls Eight Windows, NY, NY, 1996;pp.39-40.

60 Chernobyl: *Assessment of Radiological and Health Impact, 2002 Update of Chernobyl: Ten Years On*, Chapter II: The release, dispersion and deposition of radionuclide. OECD. See: http://www.oecd-nea.org/rp/chernobyl/c02.html.

61 See page 2, section 5 at: See: http://www.iaea.org/newscenter/features/chernobyl-15/cherno-faq.shtml.

62 U. S. National Cancer Institute (NCI) Withheld Atom-Bomb Test Data: Radioactive Fallout (Iodine) Increased Thyroid Cancer in U. S. : See: http://www.preventcancer.com/losing/nci/nci_atom_bomb.htm.

63 Gould JM, Sternglass EJ, Managan JJ. U.S.A. Newborn Deterioration in the Nuclear Age, 1945-1996. Presented at the International Congress on the Effects of Low-dose Ionizing Radiation in Childhood and Youth, In: *Medicine, Industry and Environment in the Workplace*. 1998 Mar 19 – 21. See: http://www.radiation.org/reading/newborn/newborn_article.html.

64 Zablotska LB, et al. A cohort study of thyroid cancer and other thyroid diseases after the Chornobyl accident: dose-response analysis of thyroid follicular adenomas detected during first screening in Ukraine (1998-2000). *Am J Epidemiol*. 2008 Feb 1;167(3):305-12.

65 Evets LV, et al. [The biological effect of low-level radiation doses on the morphological composition of the peripheral blood in children*]. Radiobiologiia*. 1992 Sep-Oct;32(5):627-31.

66 Jacob P, et al. Thyroid cancer risk in areas of Ukraine and Belarus affected by the Chernobyl accident. *Radiat Res*. 2006 Jan;165(1):1-8.

67 Starr M. Hypothyroidism Type 2. See: http://www.amazon.com/Hypothyroidism-Type-Epidemic-Mark-Starr/dp/0975262408/ref=sr_1_1?ie=UTF8&s=books&qid=1267429210&sr=8-1.

68 Gilbert ES, Tarone R, Ron E, Bouville A. Thyroid cancer rates and ^{131}I doses from Nevada atmospheric nuclear bomb tests. *J Natl Cancer Inst*. 1998;90(21):1654-60.

69 Also see: http://en.wikipedia.org/wiki/Nuclear_weapons_testing.

70 See page 2, section 5 at: See: http://www.iaea.org/newscenter/features/chernobyl-15/cherno-faq.shtml.

71 Gonzalez AJ. Radioactive Residues of the Cold War Period: A Radiological Legacy. IAEA Bulletin. 1998;40(4):3 & 5.

72 See page 4, section 12 at: See: http://www.iaea.org/newscenter/features/chernobyl-15/cherno-faq.shtml.

73 Chernobyl: Assessment of Radiological and Health Impact, 2002 Update of Chernobyl: Ten Years On, Chapter II: The release, dispersion and deposition of radionuclide. OECD. See: http://www.oecd-nea.org/rp/chernobyl/c02.html.

74 Yablokov, A. V. Nesterenko, V. B. Chernobyl Contamination through Time and Space. Ann N Y Acad Sci. 2009;1181(1):5-30.

75 Yablokov AV, Nesterenko VB, Nesterenko AV. *Chernobyl: Consequences of the Catastrophe for People and the Environment*. Chapter II. Consequences of the

Chernobyl catastrophe for public health. Section 2. Chernobyl's public health consequences – some methodological problems. *Ann N Y Acad Sci*. 2009 Dec;1181(1).

76 Yablokov AV, Nesterenko VB, Nesterenko AV. Chernobyl: *Consequences of the Catastrophe for People and the Environment*. Section 3. General Morbidity, Impairment, and Disability after the Chernobyl Catastrophe. *Ann N Y Acad Sci.* 2009 Dec;1181(1).

77 Sanderson C. Chernobyl — Out of the Darkness. *Townsend Letter*. 1993 Aug-Sep; (121/122):785.

78 See Professor Richard Day's article in the July 1st, 1991 issue of *The Pittsburg Post*, plus Dr. Alice Stewart and Dr. George Kneale's report in The New York Times, December 1992, who "present a more sinister picture of the risks of small doses of radiation."

79 Wotawa G. Accident in the Japanese NPP Fukushima: Spread of Radioactivity/weather currently not favourable (Update: 2011 Mar 25, 16:00) ZAMG – Division for Data, Methods and Modelling, Central Institute for Meteorology and Geodynamics. Hohe Warte 38, 1190 Wien.

80 Chernobyl: Assessment of Radiological and Health Impact, 2002 Update of Chernobyl: Ten Years On, Chapter II: The release, dispersion and deposition of radionuclide. OECD. See: http://www.oecd-nea.org/rp/chernobyl/c02.html.

81 See: http://www.reuters.com/article/2011/06/28/us-japan-nuclear-idUSTRE75Q1EV20110628.

82 Kilham C. Medicine Hunter Radiation in Our Food. Published June 30, 2011, FoxNews.com. See: http://www.foxnews.com/health/2011/06/29/radiation-in-our-food/.

83 See: http://www.davistownmuseum.org/cbm/Rad10.html and: http://www.epa.gov/radiation/rert/nuclearblast.html.

84 Norris RS, Chochran T, Arkin W. Known U.S. Nuclear Tests. Washington D.C.: Natural Resources Defense Council. 1988. See also Natural Resources Defense Council: Nuclear Weapons Handbook. Volume IV. New York: Harper & Row, 1989.

85 See Null G. Fatal Fallout: The Dangers of Ionizing Radiation. pages 5 & 14 at: http://029bdc8.netsolhost.com/graphics/fatalfallout.pdf.

86 See: http://www.conflict-resolution.org/sitebody/education/lecture_series/Caldicott.htm.

87 See: http://www.nytimes.com/2011/05/01/opinion/01caldicott.html.

88 Yablokov AV. 11. Chernobyl's radioactive impact on microbial biota. *Ann N Y Acad Sci.* 2009 Nov;1181(1):281-4.

89 Stewart A. A-Bomb Data: Detection of Bias in the Life Span Study Cohort. *Environ Health Perspect* 1997; 105(Suppl 6):1519-21. See: http://www.ncbi.nlm.nih.gov/pmc/articles/PMC1469934/pdf/envhper00331-0137.pdf.

90 See: http://idsc.nih.go.jp/idwr/kanja/weeklygraph/16bacmen.html.

91 See: http://idsc.nih.go.jp/idwr/kanja/weeklygraph/07parvo.html.

92 See: http://idsc.nih.go.jp/idwr/kanja/weeklygraph/06HFMD.html.

93 See: http://idsc.nih.go.jp/idwr/kanja/weeklygraph/18myco.html.

94 See: http://idsc.nih.go.jp/idwr/kanja/weeklygraph/21RSV.html.

95 See: http://idsc.nih.go.jp/idwr/ydata/report-Ja.html.

96 World Health Organization. Outbreaks of E. coli O104:H4 infection: See: http://www.euro.who.int/en/what-we-do/health-topics/emergencies/international-health-regulations/outbreaks-of-e.-coli-o104h4-infection.

97 Schneider K. Converted radioactive waste used to fertilize in Oklahoma. Special to *The New York Times.* 1987 Nov 16. See: http://www.nytimes.com/1987/11/16/us/converted-radioactive-waste-used-to-fertilize-in-oklahoma.html..

98 Nesterenko AV, Nesterenko VB, Yablokov AV. 12. Chernobyl's radioactive contamination of food and people. *Ann N Y Acad Sci.* 2009 Nov;1181:289-302.

99 Wolf I. Recycled radioactive metal contaminates consumer products. Scripps Howard News Service. 2009 Jun 3. See: http://www.scrippsnews.com/node/43577.

100 See: http://online.wsj.com/article/SB10001424052748704613504576268431769391772.html.

101 See: http://www.torontosun.com/news/world/2011/04/16/18020536.html.

102 Nuclear Expert: Radioactive Rain-Outs Will Continue For a Year – Even In Western U.S. and Canada – Because Japanese Are Burning Radioactive Materials. The Intel Hub Washington's Blog. 2011 Aug 17; see: http://theintelhub.com/2011/08/17/nuclear-expert-radioactive-rain-outs-will-continue-for-a-year-%E2%80%93-even-in-western-u-s-and-canada-%E2%80%93-because-japanese-are-burning-radioactive-materials/.

103 FDA Blocks Japanese Imports: Dr. Richard Besser takes you behind the scenes at JFK International Airport. ABC News. 2011 Mar 22. See: http://abcnews.go.com/WNT/video/fda-blocks-japanese-imports-radiation-fears-jfk-airport-richard-besser-13197729?tabID=9482930&sectionID=1206853&playlistID=13198095.

104 See: http://www.fda.gov/newsevents/publichealthfocus/ucm247403.htm.

105 Satoko N. Say-Peace Project, protecting children against radiation: citizens take radiation protection into their own hands, *The Asia-Pacific Journal*, Volume 9, Issue 25, No. 1, June 20, 2011. See: http://www.japanfocus.org/-Norimatsu-Satoko/3549.

106 See: http://enformable.com/2011/08/radioactive-beef-consumed-in-school-lunches-in-296-schools-in-12-prefectures-in-japan-ex-skf/.

107 Wing S, Richardson D, Armstrong D, Crawford-Brown D. A reevaluation of cancer incidence near the Three Mile Island Nuclear Plant: the collision of evidence and assumptions. *Environ Health Perspect.* 1997;105:52-7.

108 Hatch M, Susser M, Beyea J. Comments on "A reevaluation of cancer incidence near the Three Mile Island Nuclear Plant" [letter]. *Environ Health Perspect.* 1997;105:12.

109 Wing S, Richardson DB, Hoffmann W. Cancer risks near nuclear facilities: the importance of research design and explicit study hypotheses. *Environ Health Perspect.* 2011;119:417–21 (2011).

110 Petkau A. effect of Na-22 on phospholipid membranes. *Health Physics.*1972 Mar.

111 Pekau A. Radiation carcinogenesis from a membrane perspective. *Acta Physiol Scand.* 1980;(Suppl. 492):81-90.

112 ECRR. *Recommendations of the European Committee on Radiation Risk: Health Effects of Ionizing Radiation Exposure at Low Doses for Radiation Protection Purposes.* Green Audit Books, Aberystwyth, 2003;p.186.

113 Burlakova EB. Low intensity radiation: Radiobiological aspects. *Rad Protect Dosimet.* 1995;62(1/2):13-8.

114 Sgouros G, Knox SJ, Joiner MC, Morgan WF, Kassis AI. MIRD continuing education: Bystander and low dose-rate effects: are these relevant to radionuclide therapy? J *Nucl Med.* 2007 Oct;48(10):1683-91.

115 Asur R, Balasubramaniam M, Marples B, Thomas RA, Tucker JD. Bystander effects induced by chemicals and ionizing radiation: evaluation of changes in gene expression of downstream MAPK targets. *Mutagenesis.* 2010 May;25(3):271-9.

116 Wideł M, Przybyszewski W, Rzeszowska-Wolny J. [Radiation-induced bystander effect: the important part of ionizing radiation response. *Potential clinical implications].* *Postepy Hig Med Dosw* (Online). 2009 Aug 18;63:377-88.

117 Asur R, Balasubramaniam M, Marples B, Thomas RA, Tucker JD. Bystander effects induced by chemicals and ionizing radiation: evaluation of changes in gene expression of downstream MAPK targets. *Mutagenesis.* 2010 May;25(3):271-9.

118 Schilling-Tóth B, et al. Analysis of the common deletions in the mitochondrial DNA is a sensitive biomarker detecting direct and non-targeted cellular effects of low dose ionizing radiation. www.ncbi.nlm.nih.gov/pubmed/21843534" \ "Mutation research." 2011 Aug 5. [Epub ahead of print].

119 Ilnytskyy Y, Kovalchuk O. Non-targeted radiation effects-An epigenetic connection. *Mutat Res.* 2011 Sep 1;714(1-2):113-25.

120 Yang H, Asaad N, Held KD. Medium-mediated intercellular communication is involved in bystander responses of X-ray-irradiated normal human fibroblasts. *Oncogene.* 2005 Mar 17;24(12):2096-103.

121 Herok R, et al. Bystander effects induced by medium from irradiated cells: similar transcriptome responses in irradiated and bystander K562 cells. *Int J Radiat Oncol Biol Phys.* 2010 May 1;77(1):244-52.

122 Yang H, Asaad N, Held KD. Medium-mediated intercellular communication is involved in bystander responses of X-ray-irradiated normal human fibroblasts. *Oncogene.* 2005 Mar 17;24(12):2096-103.

123 Krick R, et al. Piecemeal microautophagy of the nucleus requires the core macroautophagy genes. *Mol Biol Cell.* 2008 Oct;19(10):4492-505.

124 Gould JA. *The Enemy Within: The High Cost of Living Near Nuclear Reactors*. Four Walls Eight Windows, NY, NY, 1996;pp.72-8.

125 Null G, et al. What Physicians Should Know About the Biological Effects of Ingested Fission Products.:812-15.

126 See #3: http://hps.org/publicinformation/ate/q6091.html.

127 Busby C. ECRR Uranium and Health: The Health Effects of Exposure to Uranium and Uranium Weapons Fallout. Documents of the ECRR 2010 No 2. Brussels, 2010;pp. 10-1.

128 See Null G. Fatal Fallout: The Dangers of Ionizing Radiation, page 21 at: http://029bdc8.netsolhost.com/graphics/fatalfallout.pdf.

129 Graeub R. *The Petkau Effect: Nuclear Radiation, People and Trees.* Four Walls Eight Windows, NY, NY, 1992;p.xxi.

130 The dispersal and penetration refers to: (A) surface area, (B) surface energy, (C) character of radioactive emissions and (D) concentrations of parent and daughter radionuclides.

131 See: http://www.nrc.gov/reading-rm/basic-ref/students/reactors.html.

132 Del Debbio JA. Removal of cesium from a high-level calcined waste by high temperature volatilization. Idaho National Engineering Laboratory. 1994 Nov;INEL-94/0028 (DOE Contract No. DE-AC07-94ID13223. See: http://www.iaea.org/inis/collection/NCLCollectionStore/_Public/27/032/27032291.pdf.

133 Lewis BJ, et al. Modelling the Release Behavior of Cesium During Severe Fuel Degradation, Table 1: Summary of vertical radiation (VI Series) tests at-ORNL; page 5B-95 (CA9800595). See: http://www.iaea.org/inis/collection/NCLCollectionStore/_Public/30/000/30000527.pdf.

134 Corradini K. Vapor Explosions: A Review of Experiments for Accident Analysis. Nuclear Safety. 1991;32(3):337-62.

135 Corradini K, Oh. Vapor Explosions in Light Water Reactors: A Review of Theory and Modeling. Progress in Nuclear Energy. 1988;22(1):1-117.

136 Corradini K. Vapor Explosions: A Review of Experiments for Accident Analysis. Nuclear Safety. 1991;32(3):337-62.

137 See: http://uk.ask.com/wiki/Zircaloy.

138 Private communication with Arnie Gundersen, October 31st, 2011.

139 Corradini K. Vapor Explosions: A Review of Experiments for Accident Analysis, Nuclear Safety, 1991;32(3):337-62. Also see: http://worldwidescience.org/topicpages/s/steam+explosion+loads.html.

140 See: http://www.infiniteunknown.net/2011/05/17/prof-chris-busby-on-rt-situation-at-fukushima-out-of-control-there-have-been-nuclear-explosions-ongoing-nuclear-reaction-taking-place-now%e2%80%9d/.

141 Gundersen A. New TEPCO Photographs Substantiate Significant Damage to Fukushima Unit 3. Fairewinds Associates – Analysis and Solutions to Complex Engineering, Environment, Energy, and Legal Issues. See: http://fairewinds.com/content/new-tepco-photographs-substantiate-significant-damage-fukushima-unit-3.

142 See: http://en.wikipedia.org/wiki/Nuclear_explosion.

143 Private communication with Arnie Gundersen, May 23rd, 2011.

144 Alvarez R, et al. Reducing the hazards from stored spent power-reactor fuel in the United States, *Science and Global Security*. 2003;11:10.

145 Takemura T, et al. A numerical simulation of global transport of atmospheric particles emitted from the Fukushima Daiichi Nuclear Power Plant. *SOLA*. 2011;7:101-4.

146 See: http://mdn.mainichi.jp/mdnnews/news/20110513p2a00m0na019000c.html.

147 YASUDA T. Report suggests second meltdown at reactor at Fukushima plant, AJW by the Asahi Shimbun, 2011 Aug 8. See: http://ajw.asahi.com/article/0311disaster/fukushima/AJ201108085674

148 After Japan Nuclear Power Plant Disaster: How Much Radioactivity in the Oceans? National Science Foundation (Press Release 11-100). 2011 May 18. See: http://www.nsf.gov/news/news_summ.jsp?org=NSF&cntn_id=119577&preview=false and the charts at: http://www.nsf.gov/news/news_images.jsp?cntn_id=119577&org=NSF.

149 Readings as high as 5M Bq/M2 verses 550K Bq/M2 25 miles out from Fukushima Daiichi compared to Chernobyl.

150 See: http://www.iaea.org/newscenter/news/2011/fukushima130411.html.

151 Chernobyl: Assessment of Radiological and Health Impact, 2002 Update of Chernobyl: Ten Years On, Chapter II: The release, dispersion and deposition of radionuclide. OECD. See: http://www.oecd-nea.org/rp/chernobyl/c02.html.

152 Gonzalez AJ. Radioactive Residues of the Cold War Period: A Radiological Legacy. *IAEA Bulletin*. 1998;40(4):3 & 5.

153 RADNET. Section 10: Chernobyl Fallout Data: Annotated Bibliography.

See: http://www.davistownmuseum.org/cbm/Rad7.html; and see: Wohni T. External doses from radioactive fallout: Dosimetry and Levels. Department of Physics, Norwegian Instituted of Technology. University of Trondheim, Norwegian Radiation Protection Authority, Oslo, 1993.

154 Napier BA. Selection of Dominant Radionuclides for Phase I of the Hanford Environmental Dose Reconstruction Project, Appendices D & E. PNL-7231 HEDR,

1991 Jul. Also see: http://hanford-downwinders.tribe.net/thread/27ac20d9-46ee-4fd7-9fae-15a0be3a7665.

155 Hanson LA. Radioactive Waste Contamination of Soil and Groundwater at the Hanford Site. University of Idaho, *Principles of Environmental Toxicology* 2000 Nov; p. 4. See: http://www.agls.uidaho.edu/etox/resources/case_studies/HANFORD.PDF. [Ref: 437 million Curies = 16,169 X 10^{15} Bq total radioactivity].

156 U.S. EPA, Environmental Radiation Protection Standards for Management and Disposal of Spent Nuclear Fuel, High-Level and Transuranic Radioactive Wastes. Table 1.4 (IDB Reference Characteristics of LWR Nuclear Fuel Assemblies). Code of Federal Regulations. 40 CFR Part 191 (July 1, 1996).

157 Borovoi AA, Sich AR. The Chernobyl accident revisited, part II: The state of the nuclear fuel located within the Chernobyl sarcophagus. *Nuclear Safety*. 1995;36(1).

158 Asano T. 3.20 Studies of Radiological Consequences on the Reports of Chernobyl Accident, JAERI Conference 99-011. IAEA INIS Collection; page 318. See: http://www.iaea.org/inis/collection/NCLCollectionStore/_Public/31/017/31017713.pdf#search=JAERI-Conf 99-011.

159 Fukushima Daiichi Nuclear Power Station: Analysis Results of Spent Fuel Pool Water in Unit 1 to 4. TEPCO 2011 Aug 25; see: http://www.tepco.co.jp/en/nu/fukushima-np/images/handouts_110825_02-e.pdf

160 As reported by Japan's Ministry of Economy, Trade and Industry, March 17th, 2011. See Fukushima Nuclear Accident Update, March 22nd, 2011, 18:00 UTC: http://www.iaea.org/newscenter/news/2011/fukushima220311.html.

161 TEPCO confirms damage to part of No. 4 unit's spent nuke fuel. Kyodo News. Tokyo 2011 Apr 11. See: http://english.kyodonews.jp/news/2011/04/85295.html.

162 Takahara K. Radiation surges above 4's fuel pool. The Japan Times. 2011 Apr 14. See: http://search.japantimes.co.jp/cgi-bin/nn20110414a1.html.

163 Core Meltdown on Fresh Air, Nearly no retention of fission products, large released: The Fukushima Daiichi Incident – Dr. Matthias Braun – 7 April 2011 © AREVA 2011; pages 31-2.

164 As reported by Japan's Ministry of Economy, Trade and Industry, March 17th, 2011. See Fukushima Nuclear Accident Update, March 22nd, 2011, 18:00 UTC: http://www.iaea.org/newscenter/news/2011/fukushima220311.html.

165 Dr.-Ing. Ludger Mohrbach, Linnemann T, Schäfer G, Vallana G. Earthquake and Tsunami in Japan on March 11, 2011 and Consequences for Fukushima and other Nuclear Power Plants, Status: April 15, 2011.VGB PowerTech e.V.; Slide 60. See: www.vgb.org.

166 Ryall J. Nuclear fuel has melted through base of Fukushima plant. The Telegraph. UK, 2011 Jun 9, 1:06AM BST.

167 As reported by Japan's Ministry of Economy, Trade and Industry, March 17th, 2011. See Fukushima Nuclear Accident Update, March 22nd, 2011, 18:00 UTC: http://www.iaea.org/newscenter/news/2011/fukushima220311.html.

168 Japan Reactor's Spent Fuel Storage Heating Up. CBC News. 2011 Mar 22nd, 7:53AM. See: http://news.aol.ca/2011/03/22/japan-reactors-spent-fuel-storage-heating-up/19887449.

169Dr.-Ing. Ludger Mohrbach, Linnemann T, Schäfer G, Vallana G. Earthquake and Tsunami in Japan on March 11, 2011 and Consequences for Fukushima and other Nuclear Power Plants, Status: April 15, 2011.VGB PowerTech e.V.; Slide 60. See: www.vgb.org.

170 Ryall J. Nuclear fuel has melted through base of Fukushima plant. *The Telegraph*. UK, 2011 Jun 9, 1:06AM BST.

171 As reported by Japan's Ministry of Economy, Trade and Industry. 2011 Mar 17th. See Fukushima Nuclear Accident Update, 2011 Mar 22nd, 18:00 UTC: http://www.iaea.org/newscenter/news/2011/fukushima220311.html.

172Dr.-Ing. Ludger Mohrbach, Linnemann T, Schäfer G, Vallana G. Earthquake and Tsunami in Japan on March 11, 2011 and Consequences for Fukushima and other Nuclear Power Plants, Status: April 15, 2011.VGB PowerTech e.V.; Slide 60. See: www.vgb.org.

173 Ryall J. Nuclear fuel has melted through base of Fukushima plant. *The Telegraph*. UK, 2011 Jun 9, 1:06AM BST.

174 Epidemiologists are bound to debate this comparison for an extended period of time, since the radiation accumulation per square meter or per square kilometer is still rising as of this writing. For now, a gross estimate could be based on the population of these respective regions per square kilometer. Japan's population per square kilometer is ~337 persons living within 1 square kilometer (see: http://en.wikipedia.org/wiki/Demographics_of_Japan). The greater Chernobyl region (Ukraine, Belarus and the Bryansk region of Russia) has a mean of ~57 persons living within 1 square kilometer (Ukraine = ~80/km2, Belarus ~50/km2 & Bryansk region ~40/km2). See: http://www.kosivart.com/eng/index.cfm/do/ukraine.population/;http://countrystudies.us/belarus/17.htm; and, http://www.vostok.cc/city.php?id=24 respectively.

175 Speaking at a C-Span press conference on March 25, 2011, in Washington, DC, Dr. Alexey Yablokov (co-author of "Chernobyl: Consequences of the Catastrophe for People and the Environment," and a member of the Russian Academy of Sciences), said: "We are seeing something that has never happened – a multiple reactor catastrophe including one using plutonium fuel as well as spent fuel pool accidents, all happening within 200 kilometers of a metropolis of 30 million people. Because the area is far more densely populated than around Chernobyl, the human toll could eventually be far worse in Japan." See conference on C-Span at: http://www.c-spanvideo.org/program/Chernob.

176 See: http://www.nuc.berkeley.edu/node/4151.

177 See Dispersion and Deposition of Chernobyl Fallout: http://www.nukefree.org/news/theotherchernobylreport.

178 See: http://www.iaea.org/newscenter/news/2011/fukushima200511.html.

179 Ukraine's most contaminated region was populated by 2.6 million people at the time of the catastrophe.

180 5 million most affected. See: http://faculty.virginia.edu/metals/cases/kleinfeld3.html.

181 25% of Belarus' 10 million citizens were contaminated at the time of the catastrophe, or 2.5 million people See: http://uecb.by.ru/eng/belarus/chernobyl1.htm.

182 Humber Y, Biggs S. Fukushima risks Chernobyl 'dead zone.' Bloomberg. 2011 May 30. See: http://www.bloomberg.com/news/2011-05-30/japan-risks-chernobyl-like-dead-zone-as-fukushima-soil-radiation-soars.html.

183 Hirsch H. Fukushima – INES scale rating. Greenpeace International. 2011 Mar 23. See: http://www.greenpeace.org/usa/PageFiles/285414/greenpeace_hirsch_INES_report_25032011.pdf.

184 Bowyer TW, et al. Elevated radioxenon detected remotely following the Fukushima nuclear accident. *J Environ Radioact*. 2011 Jul;102(7):681-7.

185 Personal email communication from Arnie Gundersen, chief nuclear engineer at Fairewinds.com, August 13th, 2011.

186 Fukushima Failures kept behind closed doors at IAEA Meeting. Bloomberg *Business Week*. 2011 Jun 20. See: http://news.businessweek.com/article.asp?documentKey=1376-LN2BLU1A1I4H01-51O4KU6OVMMLHQ96S0QGJE0R5O.

187 See: http://fairewinds.com/content/newly-released-tepco-data-proves-fairewinds-assertions-significant-fuel-pool-failures-fukush.

188 See: http://www.nytimes.com/2011/07/30/science/earth/30radiation.html?_r=1.

189 McGarity TO, Wager WE. *Bending Science: How Special Interests Corrupt Public Health Research*. Harvard University Press, Cambridge, MA, 2008;pp.34-6.

190 See: http://www.nuc.berkeley.edu/node/2371.

191 See: http://www.nuc.berkeley.edu/node/2371.

192 See: http://edi-nm.com/about_us.htm.

193 See page 5: https://www.gsaadvantage.gov/ref_text/GS10F0341R/0ED012.1P4SM7_GS-10F-0341R_EDIPROFILERATESREV1.PDF

194 Bowyer, et al. Elevated radioxenon detected remotely following the Fukushima nuclear accident. *Journal of Environmental Radioactivity* 2011 Jul;102(7):681-7.

195 See: http://www.epa.gov/japan2011/rert/radnet-seattle-bg.html#air

196 Masamichi N. The Problem of radiation exposure countermeasures for the Fukushima nuclear accident: concerns for the present situation. *Toyo Keizai*. 2011 Jun 27. See: http://japanfocus.org/events/view/100?rand=1309582023&type=print&print=1.

197 FOIA Document # ML11244A169, pp. 167-9. See: http://enformable.com/2011/10/the-nrc-knew-possibility-of-elevated-thyroid-

dose-in-midway-island-and-alaska-by-march-22nd-worked-to-keep-it-away-from-foia/.

198 Email From Mike Franovich, NRC Technical Assistant for Reactors, sent Thursday, March 24th, 2011 at 7:20AM, to NRC Commissioner William Ostendorff, Subject: UPDATE from 200 Telecon on Fukushima Daiichi Events, p. 38 (marked at bottom of page as p. 48). See: http://pbadupws.nrc.gov/docs/ML1124/ML11244A210.pdf

199 See: http://www.epa.gov/japan2011/rert/radnet-sacramento-bg.html.

200 See: http://www.nuc.berkeley.edu/node/2371.

201One atmosphere = ~14.7 pounds per square inch at sea level See: http://en.wikipedia.org/wiki/Atmospheric_pressure.

202 Dr.-Ing. Ludger Mohrbach, Linnemann T, Schäfer G, Vallana G. Earthquake and Tsunami in Japan on March 11, 2011 and Consequences for Fukushima and other Nuclear Power Plants, Status: April 15, 2011.VGB PowerTech e.V.; Slide 60. See: www.vgb.org.

203 Yasuda T. Report suggests second meltdown at reactor at Fukushima plant, AJW by the Asahi Shimbun, 2011 Aug 8. See: http://ajw.asahi.com/article/0311disaster/fukushima/AJ201108085674.

204 See the National Oceanic & Atmospheric Administration (NOAA): http://www.ncdc.noaa.gov/sotc/hazards/2011/3.

205 See the Google Charts at: http://pstuph.wordpress.com/2011/04/04/epas-radnet-troubles/.

206 See: http://www.ncdc.noaa.gov/sotc/hazards/2011/4.

207 See: http://www.doh.wa.gov/ehp/rp/rep/aerial.htm.

208 See: http://blogs.forbes.com/jeffmcmahon/2011/04/27/radioactive-strontium-found-in-hilo-hawaii-milk/.

209 See: http://www.epa.gov/radiation/docs/rert/radnet-cart-filter-final.pdf.

210 See: http://blogs.forbes.com/jeffmcmahon/2011/04/09/radiation-detected-in-drinking-water-in-13-more-us-cities-cesium-137-in-vermont-milk/.

211 See: http://www.nsf.gov/news/news_summ.jsp?org=NSF&cntn_id=119577&preview=false.

212 See the National Science Foundation article: http://www.nsf.gov/news/news_images.jsp?cntn_id=119577&org=NSF.

213 See: http://blogs.forbes.com/jeffmcmahon/2011/05/17/scientists-will-use-fukushima-radiation-to-study-ocean-currents/.

214 See the National Science Foundation article: http://www.nsf.gov/news/news_images.jsp?cntn_id=119577&org=NSF.

215 See Figure 1 in: Priyadarshi A, Dominguez G, Thiemens MH. Evidence of neutron leakage at the Fukushima nuclear plant from measurements of radioactive 35S in California. *Proc Natl Acad Sci.* 2011 Aug 15. See: www.pnas.org/cgi/doi/10.1073/pnas.1109449108.

216 Vancouver seaweed almost 400% above international limit for iodine-131 in food... by March 28 — Levels increasing. ENEWS. 2011 Apr 5,t 09:34 PM. See: http://enenews.com/vancouver-seaweed-almost-400-above-international-standard-for-iodine-131-in-food-by-march-28-levels-increasing.

217 See: http://sirocco.omp.obs-mip.fr/outils/Symphonie/Produits/Japan/SymphoniePreviJapan.htm.

218 Winiarek V, Bocquet M, Roustan Y, Birman C, Tran P. Atmospheric dispersion of radionuclides from the Fukushima-Daichii nuclear power plant: Map of ground deposition of caesium-137 for the Fukushima-Daichii accident, CEREA, joint laboratory École des Ponts ParisTech and EdF R&D. See: http://cerea.enpc.fr/fr/fukushima.html.

219 Also see the full animation at: http://enformable.com/2011/09/france-releases-map-of-cesium-137-deposition-across-the-pacific-shows-the-us-more-contaminated-than-western-japan-ex-skf/.

220 See: Http://www.yomiuri.co.jp/science/news/20110719-OYT1T01036.htm?from=main2.

221 Cesium in incinerator dust across east Japan. The Japan Times Online. Kyodo, 2011 Aug 29; see: http://search.japantimes.co.jp/cgi-bin/nn20110829a5.html.

222 See: http://www.mext.go.jp/english/incident/1303986.htm.

223 See: http://www.tpub.com/content/chemical-biological/TM-1-1500-335-23/css/TM-1-1500-335-23_659.htm.

224 See: http://www.epa.gov/radon/healthrisks.html.

225 Makhijani A. Fukushima Fallout Monitoring Needed. 2011 Apr 8. See: http://www.ieer.org/comments/FukushimaFallout_in_US_20110407.html.

226 Health Risks from Exposure to Low Levels of Ionizing Radiation: BEIR VII – Phase 2 Committee to Assess Health Risks from Exposure to Low Levels of Ionizing Radiation. National Research Council. For free download see: http://www.nap.edu/catalog/11340.html.

227 NRC: National Research Council (2005). Biologic effects of ionizing radiation VII: Health risks from exposure to low levels of ionizing radiation. National Academy of Science. Washington DC. See: http://www.nirs.org/press/06-30-2005/1.

228 See: http://www.fpl.com/environment/nuclear/nukebook_measuring_radiation.shtml.

229 See: http://www.prisonplanet.com/dangerous-levels-of-radiation-recorded-in-canada-as-fukushima-radiation-dangers-continue.html and see: http://www.youtube.com/watch?v=dccszCEKFdY.

230 See: http://www.epa.gov/radnet00/images/beta-gamma/sacramento-beta.jpg.

231 See: http://www.nuc.berkeley.edu/node/3001.

232 See: http://www.epa.gov/japan2011/rert/radnet-sampling-data.html.

233 See: http://www.nuc.berkeley.edu/RainWaterSampling.

234 Also see: http://enenews.com/radioactive-iodine-131-in-rainwater-sample-near-san-francisco-is-18100-above-federal-drinking-water-standard.

235 See: http://midsurreylink.org/chernobyl.

236 For solutions also see: http://www.dairyherd.com/dairy-news/latest/Effects-of-Radiation-on-Food-Animals-118360969.html.

237 See: http://www.nuc.berkeley.edu/node/2174.

238 See: http://blogs.forbes.com/jeffmcmahon/2011/04/27/radioactive-strontium-found-in-hilo-hawaii-milk/.

239 Health Risks from Exposure to Low Levels of Ionizing Radiation: BEIR VII – Phase 2 Committee to Assess Health Risks from Exposure to Low Levels of Ionizing Radiation. National Research Council. For free download see: http://www.nap.edu/catalog/11340.html.

240 NRC: National Research Council (2005). Biologic effects of ionizing radiation VII: Health risks from exposure to low levels of ionizing radiation. National Academy of Science. Washington DC. See: http://www.nirs.org/press/06-30-2005/1.

241 See: http://dictionary.reference.com/browse/bioaccumulate.

242 Chapter II: The release, dispersion and deposition of radionuclides – Chernobyl: Assessment of Radiological and Health Impact, 2002 Update on Chernobyl: Ten Years On. See: http://www.oecd-nea.org/rp/chernobyl/c02.html.

243 Table 3: Evolution of average radioactivity in the Pripiat river since the accident in 1986 (From Poikaprpov and Robeau, 2001), Chapter II, Ibid. See: http://www.oecd-nea.org/rp/chernobyl/c02.html.

244 See: http://www.spiegel.de/international/zeitgeist/0,1518,709345,00.html.

245 See: http://www.bbc.co.uk/news/science-environment-10819027.

246 See: http://www.nytimes.com/2010/08/11/world/europe/11russia.html.

247 See: http://www.ens-newswire.com/ens/apr2010/2010-04-26-01.html.

248 Post-Chernobyl Thyroid Disease in the United States of America by Jay M. Gould, Ernest J. Sternglass and Joseph J. Mangano, presented to The International Medical Commission Conference: Chernobyl: Environmental Health and Human Rights Implications (Vienna, April 12-15, 1996), RPHP Series 1, Number 1. See: http://www.radiation.org/reading/index.html.

249 Gould JM, Sternglass EJ. Low-level radiation and mortality. *Chemtech*, American Chemical Society. 1989 Jan.

250 Mangano JJ, Reid W. Thyroid cancer in America since Chernobyl. *BMJ*. 1995 Aug;303(7003):511.

251 Mangano JJ. A post-Chernobyl rise in Connecticut thyroid cancer. *Europena Journal of Cancer Prevention.* 1996 Jan;5(1).

252 Scholz, R. Ten Years After Chernobyl: The Rise of Strontium-90 In Baby Teeth. Munich. Introduction by Jay M. Gould, RPHP Series 1, Number 5. See: http://www.radiation.org/reading/index.html/.

253 McMahon J. EPA Halts Extra Radiation Monitoring; Focus Shifts To Imported Seafood. Forbes. 2011 May 04 @ 9:26AM. See: http://www.forbes.com/sites/jeffmcmahon/2011/05/04/epa-halts-extra-radiation-monitoring-focus-shifts-to-seafood/.

254 Canada suspends mobile radiation measurements around Vancouver, BC "until further notice" as radioactive cloud looms (VIDEO). ENEWS. April 4th, 2011 at 06:46 AM. See: http://enenews.com/canada-suspends-mobile-radiation-measurements-around-vancouver-bc-further-notice.

255 See: https://docs.google.com/document/pub?id=1e0VxH-YSMw7dRlrVpmi69jpCWrwn8k1f0T2gZWWG73Q.

256 See: http://blog.alexanderhiggins.com/2011/04/21/radioactive-fukushima-plutonium-strontium-bombarding-west-coast-march-18th-19279/.

257 Leon JD, et al. Nuclear Experiment: Arrival time and magnitude of airborne fission products from the Fukushima, Japan, reactor incident as measured in Seattle, WA, USA, Cornell University Library (Submitted on 24 Mar 2011 (v1), last revised 25 Mar 2011 (this version, v2)), arXiv.org > nucl-ex > arXiv:1103.4853. See: http://www.technologyreview.com/blog/arxiv/26571/ which found radioactive Cesium-137/134, Iodide-133/132/131, and Tellurium-132 likely arriving from Fukushima Fall-Out landing in Seattle, WA.

258 See: http://transport.nilu.no/browser/fpv_fuku?fpp=conccol_Xe-133_;region=NH.

259 EPA RadNet Air Filter and Air Cartridge Results. EPA. 2011 Apr 6.

260 Durakovic A. Medical effects of internal contamination with uranium. *Croatian Medical Journal*. 1999;40(1):49-66.

261 Yablokov AV, Nesterenko VB, Nesterenko AV. Chernobyl: Consequences of the Catastrophe for People and the Environment. *Ann N Y Acad Sci.* 2009 Dec;1181(1):43-4, 58, 62, 68, 79-84, 161-211.

262 Jam-packed spent fuel pools raise safety questions at region's nuclear plants, Submitted by NUCBIZ on April 1, 2011 – 09:40. Professional Reactor Operator Society. See: http://www.nucpros.com/content/jam-packed-spent-fuel-pools-raise-safety-questions-regions-nuclear-plants.

263 Yablokov AV, Nesterenko VB, Nesterenko AV. Chernobyl: Consequences of the Catastrophe for People and the Environment. *Ann N Y Acad Sci*. 2009 Dec;1181(1):83-7.

264 2010 Recommendations of the ECRR: The Health Effects of Exposure to Low Doses of Ionizing Radiation. Regulator's Edition, edited by Chris Busby, with Rosalie Bertell, Inge Schmitz-Feuerhake, Molly Scott Cato and Alexey Yablokov, Published on behalf of the European Committee on Radiation Risk. Green Audit. 2010;pp.9 -11, 124-7 & 173.

265 Yablokov AV, Nesterenko VB, Nesterenko AV. Chernobyl: Consequences of the Catastrophe for People and the Environment. *Ann N Y Acad Sci.* 2009 Dec;1181(1).

266 Busby C. ECRR Uranium and Health: The Health Effects of Exposure to Uranium and Uranium Weapons Fallout. Documents of the ECRR 2010 No 2. Brussels, 2010;pp. 10-1.

267 Jacob P, et al. Thyroid cancer risk in areas of Ukraine and Belarus affected by the Chernobyl accident. Radiat Res. 2006 Jan;165(1):1-8.

268 In the nuclei of stable atoms, such as those of lead, the force binding the protons and neutrons to each other individually is great enough to hold together each nucleus as a whole. In other atoms, especially heavy ones such as those of uranium, this energy is insufficient, and the nuclei are unstable. An unstable nucleus spontaneously emits particles and energy in a process known as radioactive decay. The term radioactivity refers to the particles emitted. When enough particles and energy have been emitted to create a new, stable nucleus (often the nucleus of an entirely different element), radioactivity ceases. Uranium 238, a very unstable element, goes through 18 stages of decay before becoming a stable isotope of lead (lead 206). Some of the intermediate stages include the heavier elements thorium, radium, radon, and polonium. All known elements with atomic numbers greater than 83 (bismuth) are radioactive, and many isotopes of elements with lower atomic numbers are also radioactive. When the nuclei of isotopes that are not naturally radioactive are bombarded with high-energy particles, the result is artificial radioisotopes that decay in the same manner as natural isotopes. Each element remains radioactive for a characteristic length of time, ranging from mere microseconds to billions of years. An element's rate of decay is called its half-life. This refers to the average length of time it takes for half of its nuclei to decay. The American Heritage® Science Dictionary Copyright © 2005 by Houghton Mifflin Company. Published by Houghton Mifflin Company. All rights reserved.

269 See: http://www.nucleonica.net/wiki/index.php/Help:Decay_Engine.

270 See: http://www.ndt-ed.org/EducationResources/HighSchool/Radiography/halflife2.htm.

271 See: http://www.absoluteastronomy.com/topics/Radioactive_decay.

272 See #2: http://hps.org/publicinformation/ate/q6091.html.

273 Caldicott H. Internal Radioactive Emitters – Invisible, Tasteless, and Odorless, 2011 Jul 18. See: http://www.helencaldicott.com/?s=Internal+emitters+tasteless.

274 See: http://www.bionity.com/en/encyclopedia/Fission_product.html.

275 The tooth fairy comes to Britain. *The Ecologist*. 2000;30(3):14.

276 See: http://www.radiation.org/reading/RadioactiveBabyTeethChapter.html.

277 See: http://mdn.mainichi.jp/mdnnews/news/20110513p2g00m0dm008000c.html.

278 See: http://investmentwatchblog.com/estimating-radioactive-contamination-from-the-accident-at-fukushima-daiichi-nuclear-plant/.

279 See: http://www.fairewinds.com/content/3-2011-areva-fukushima-report.

280 The Fukushima Daiichi Incident – Dr. Matthias Braun – 7 April 2011 © AREVA 2011; pp. 17-9.

281 See: http://www.reuters.com/article/2011/06/16/idUS226115285920110616.

282 See: http://www.houseoffoust.com/fukushima/r4stability.html.

283 See page IV-31 at: http://www.iaea.org/newscenter/focus/fukushima/japan-report/chapter-4.pdf.

284 See: http://www.globalpost.com/dispatch/news/regions/asia-pacific/japan/110710/japan-earthquake-tsunami-warning.

285 See the April 6th video at the 6:58 mark: http://www.fairewinds.com/updates.

286 See: http://english.aljazeera.net/indepth/features/2011/06/201161664828302638.html.

287 McMahon J. Radiation Detected In Drinking Water In 13 More US Cities, Cesium-137 In Vermont Milk. Forbes. 4/09/2011 @ 8:15AM. See: http://www.forbes.com/sites/jeffmcmahon/2011/04/09/radiation-detected-in-drinking-water-in-13-more-us-cities-cesium-137-in-vermont-milk/.

288 See: http://healthvermont.gov/enviro/rad/japan2011.aspx.

289 Mangano J. Infant deaths soar 35% in Pacific Northwest – Area hit hardest by Japanese nuclear fallout, Radiation and Public Health Project, Ocean City, NJ, 2011 Jun 7. See: www.radiation.org.

290 Caldicott H. Internal Radioactive Emitters – Invisible, Tasteless, and Odorless. 2011 Jul 18. See: http://www.helencaldicott.com/?s=Internal+emitters+tasteless.

291 See: www.rphp.org.

292 See: http://www.youtube.com/watch?v=sMV4p6RS1c8&feature=share.

293 See: http://www.vancouversun.com/health/Spike+sudden+infant+deaths+spurs+concerns/5052290/story.html.

294 Clark JU, McFarland VA. Assessing Bioaccumulation in Aquatic Organisms Exposed to Contaminated Sediments. Miscellaneous Paper D-91-2 (1991), Environmental Laboratory, Waterways Experiment Station. Vicksburg, MS.

295 Vanderplog HA, et al. Bioaccumulation Factors for Radionuclides in Freshwater Biota. *ORNL-5002 (1975).* Environmental Sciences Division Publication, Number 783, Oak Ridge National Laboratory, Oak Ridge, TN.

296 See video of Dr. Steven Wing on April 21st : http://www.fairewinds.com/updates.

297 Yablokov AV, Nesterenko VB, Nesterenko AV. Chernobyl: Consequences of the Catastrophe for People and the Environment. *Ann N Y Acad Sci.* 2009 Dec;1181(1).

298 Raeaef LC, et al. Effective dose and time-integrated effective dose to humans from internal contamination of {sup 134}Cs and {sup 137}Cs: Results from a compilation of a Swedish national database of internal body burden of radiocaesium in various populations between 1964 and 2002, 2003 Jun 1. This study was a compilation of data on the whole-body burden of 134Cs, 137Cs and 40K in various Swedish populations between 1964 and 2002 has been made. The compilation was carried out in co-operation with the Department of Radiation Physics in Malmoe, the

Swedish Radiation Protection Authority (SSI), the Swedish Defence Research Agency Department (FOI) and the Department of Radiation Physics, Goeteborg University. See: http://worldwidescience.org/topicpages/r/radiocaesium+fallout+behaviour.html

299 Watson WS, et al. Radionuclides in seals and porpoises in the coastal waters around the UK. *Sci Total Environ*. 1999 Aug 30;234(1-3):1-13.

300 Yablokov AV, Nesterenko VB, Nesterenko AV. Chernobyl: consequences of the catastrophe for people and the environment. *Ann N Y Acad Sci.* (paperback ed.) 2009 Dec;1181(1). Wiley-Blackwell..

301 See: http://www.youtube.com/watch?v=R7JvuUwpq40.

302 2010 Recommendations of the ECRR: The Health Effects of Exposure to Low Doses of Ionizing Radiation, Regulator's Edition, Edited by Chris Busby with Rosalie Bertell, Inge Schmitz-Feuerhake, Molly Scott Cato and Alexey Yablokov, Green Audit Press, Castle Cottage, Aberystwyth, SY23 1DZ, UK, 2010. See: www.euradcom.org.

303 Wing S, Richardson D, Armstrong D, Crawford-Brown D. A reevaluation of cancer incidence near the Three Mile Island Nuclear Plant: the collision of evidence and assumptions. *Environ Health Perspect*. 105:52-57 (1997).

304 Wing S, Richardson DB, Hoffmann W. Cancer risks near nuclear facilities: the importance of research design and explicit study hypotheses. *Environ Health Perspect*. 2011;119:417–21.

305 Note 2011-05: Fukushima and radiation protection policy. *Isotopics Nuclear Consultancy*. 2011 Aug 24;pp. 1-4. See: www.isotopics.nl.

306 Busby C, Bramhall R. Is there an excess of childhood cancer in North Wales on the Menai Strait, Gwynedd? Concerns about the accuracy of analyses carried out by the Wales Cancer Intelligence Unit and those using its data. Green Audit Aberystwyth. Occasional Paper 2005/3, Nov 5th 2005;p. 19.

307 Busby C. *Health effects of low-level radiation*. BNES, Green Audit, Aberystwyth, UK 2002.

308 Dupre D. Government agreed to downplay Fukushima radiation. *The National, Human Rights Examiner*. 2011 Aug 14. See: http://www.examiner.com/human-rights-in-national/radiating-americans-with-fukushima-rain-food-secret-clinton-pact.

309 Fukushima Failures Kept Behind Closed Doors at IAEA Meeting. Bloomberg. 2011 Jun 20; See: http://news.businessweek.com/article.asp?documentKey=1376-LN2BLU1A1I4H01-51O4KU6OVMMLHQ96S0QGJE0R5O

310 Kosako T. 20 Millisieverts for Children and Kosako Toshiso's Resignation, *The Asia-Pacific Journal: Japan Focus*. 2011 May 01; translated by Tanaka Izumi. See: http://japanfocus.org/events/view/83?utm_medium=twitter&utm_source=twitterfeed.

311 Private communication with Arnie Gundersen, August 29th, 2011. NISA Mentions "Neptunium-239" in August 29 Press Conference, 2011 Aug 28: The Nuclear and Industrial Safety Agency (NISA)'s daily press conference is ongoing (August 29). The

NISA spokesman Moriyama mentions neptunium-239's conversion ratio to plutonium-239 as 1 to 1. According to the June 6 estimate by the NISA:

Plutonium-239: 3.2×10^9

Neptunium-239: 7.6×10^13

So, now (as of August 29) it is:

Plutonium-239: 7.6 x 10^13, or 76,000,000,000,000 or 76 terabecquerels

The amount of plutonium-239 has increased 23,000-fold. On August 15 I wrote about neptunium-239, half life of about 2 days, having been detected in large quantity in Iitate-mura, 35 kilometers from Fukushima I Nuclear Power Plant. I had to take down the second post on the subject, but the information was correct. Now, NISA is suddenly mentioning neptunium-239. Admission of wide dispersion of this nuclide and resultant plutonium-239 may be finally forthcoming, after more than 5 months.

312 Expert urges higher radiation exposure limit to be set for Fukushima, *Kyodo*. Tokyo, 2011 Aug 23. See: http://english.kyodonews.jp/news/2011/08/110456.html.

313 Fukushima Evacuation Zone areas uninhabitable, PM to apologize, majiroxnews, 2011 Aug 21. See: http://www.majiroxnews.com/2011/08/21/fukushima-evacuation-zone-areas-uninhabitable-pm-to-apologize/.

314 After Fukushima: nuclear dirty tricks: After nearly half a century of producing nuclear power, Japan has finally separated regulation from promotion, *The Guardian*. 2011 Aug 16; see: http://www.guardian.co.uk/commentisfree/2011/aug/16/editorial-fukushima-nuclear-dirty-tricks?INTCMP=SRCH.

315 McNeill D. Why the Fukushima disaster is worse than Chernobyl: Japan has been slow to admit the scale of the meltdown. But now the truth is coming out. *The Independent*. 2011 Aug 29. See: http://tinyurl.com/3fka982.

316 Graeub R. *The Petkau Effect: Nuclear Radiation, People and Trees*. Four Walls Eight Windows, NY, 1992.

317 Mangano JJ. Childhood leukemia in US may have risen due to fall out from Chernobyl. *BMJ*. 1997 Apr 19;314(7088):1200.

318 Wing S, Richardson DB, Hoffmann W. Cancer risks near nuclear facilities: the importance of research design and explicit study hypotheses. *Environ Health Perspect*. 2011 Apr;119(4):417-21.

319 Busby C, Bramhall R. Is there an excess of childhood cancer in North Wales on the Menai Strait, Gwynedd? Concerns about the accuracy of analyses carried out by the Wales Cancer Intelligence Unit and those using its data. Green Audit Aberystwyth. Occasional Paper. 2005/3, Nov 5th 2005;p. 19.

320 Yablokov AV, Nesterenko VB, Nesterenko AV. Chernobyl: consequences of the catastrophe for people and the environment. *Ann N Y Acad Sci*. 2009 Dec;1181(1).

321 Raeaef LC, et al. Effective dose and time-integrated effective dose to humans from internal contamination of {sup 134}Cs and {sup 137}Cs: Results from a compilation of a Swedish national database of internal body burden of radiocaesium in various populations between 1964 and 2002, 2003 Jun 1. This study was a compilation of

data on the whole-body burden of 134Cs, 137Cs and 40K in various Swedish populations between 1964 and 2002 has been made. The compilation was carried out in co-operation with the Department of Radiation Physics in Malmoe, the Swedish Radiation Protection Authority (SSI), the Swedish Defence Research Agency Department (FOI) and the Department of Radiation Physics, Goeteborg University. See: http://worldwidescience.org/topicpages/r/radiocaesium+fallout+behaviour.html.

322 Watson WS, et al. Radionuclides in seals and porpoises in the coastal waters around the UK. *Sci Total Environ*. 1999 Aug 30;234(1-3):1-13.

323 Graeub R. *The Petkau Effect: Nuclear Radiation, People and Trees*, Four Walls Eight Windows, NY, 1992.

324 Gould JA. *The Enemy Within: The High Cost of Living Near Nuclear Reactors*. Four Walls Eight Windows, NY, NY, 1996;pp.39-40 & 131.

325 Mangano JJ. Childhood leukemia in US may have risen due to Fall Out from Chernobyl. *BMJ*. 1997 Apr 19;314(7088):1200.

326 Weinberg HS, et al. Very high mutation rate in offspring of Chernobyl accident liquidators. *Proc Biol Sci*. 2001 May 22;268(1471):1001-5.

327 Busby C. *The Health Effects of Exposure to Uranium and Uranium Weapons Fallout*. ECRR Uranium and Health, Documents of the ECRR. 2010;(2), Brussels, 2010.

328 Yablokov AV, Nesterenko VB, Nesterenko AV. Chernobyl: consequences of the catastrophe for people and the environment. *Ann N Y Acad Sci*. 2009 Dec;1181(1).

329 Busby C, Bramhall R. Is there an excess of childhood cancer in North Wales on the Menai Strait, Gwynedd? Concerns about the accuracy of analyses carried out by the Wales Cancer Intelligence Unit and those using its data. Green Audit Aberystwyth. Occasional Paper. 2005/3, Nov 5th 2005;p. 19.

330 Ryabokon NI, Goncharova RI. Transgenerational accumulation of radiation damage in small mammals chronically exposed to Chernobyl fallout. *Radiat Environ Biophys*. 2006 Sep;45(3):167-77.

331 Walker JS. *Permissible Dose: A History of Radiation Protection in the Twentieth Century*. University of California Press, Berkeley, CA, 2000;pp. 140-3.

332 Kuiru A, et al. Hereditary minisatellite mutations among the offspring of Estonian Chernobyl cleanup workers. *Radiat Res*. 2003 May;159(5):651-5.

333 Weinberg HS, et al. Very high mutation rate in offspring of Chernobyl accident liquidators. *Proc Biol Sci*. 2001 May 22;268(1471):1001-5.

334 Yablokov AV, Nesterenko VB, Nesterenko AV. Chernobyl: consequences of the catastrophe for people and the environment. *Ann N Y Acad Sci*. 2009 Dec;1181(1).

335 Busby C, Bramhall R. Is there an excess of childhood cancer in North Wales on the Menai Strait, Gwynedd? Concerns about the accuracy of analyses carried out by the Wales Cancer Intelligence Unit and those using its data. Green Audit Aberystwyth. Occasional Paper. 2005/3, Nov 5th 2005;p. 19.

336 Committee on Medical Aspects of Radiation in the Environment (COMARE). *Parents occupationally exposed to radiation prior to the conception of their children. A*

review of the evidence concerning the incidence of cancer in their children. Seventh Report. Chairman: Professor B A Bridges OBE, Produced by the National Radiological Protection Board, Crown Copyright 2002.

337 See: http://doctorapsley.com/default.aspx.

338 Next, see: http://doctorapsley.com/FourPillars.aspx.

339 Finally, carefully consider the following guidelines for life: http://doctorapsley.com/GettingStarted.aspx.

340 Schechter SR. *Fighting Radiation with Foods, Herbs & Vitamins*. East-West Health Books, Brookline, MA, p. 6, 85-86.

341 Schechter SR. *Fighting Radiation with Foods, Herbs & Vitamins*. East-West Health Books, Brookline, MA, p. 6, 85-86.

342 Akizuki S. *Health Condition and Diet*. Kurie press, 1980. In: Watanabe H. Miso and its biological effects. *Research Institute for Radiation Biology and Medicine*. Hiroshima University, 1-2-3 Kasumi, Kasumi1-2-3, Minami-ku, Hiroshima, Japan, 734-8553. See: http://yufoundation.org/watanabe.pdf.

343 Ohara M, et al. Radioprotective effects of miso (fermented soy bean paste) against radiation in B6C3F1 mice: increased small intestinal crypt survival, crypt lengths and prolongation of average time to death. *Hiroshima J Med Sci*. 2001 Dec;50(4):83-6.

344 Koratkar R, Rao AV. Effect of soya bean saponines on azoxymethane-induced preneoplastic lesions in the colon of mice. *Nutr Cancer*. 1997;27: 206-9.

345 Ito A, Watanabe H, Basaran N. Effects of soy products in reducing risk of spontaneous and neutron-induced liver-tumors in mice. *Int J Oncol*. 1993 May;2(5):773-6.

346 Calvelev VL, et al. Genistein can mitigate the effect of radiation on rat lung tissue. *Radiat Res*. 2010 May;173(5):602-11.

347 Watanabe H, et al. Protection against hypertension by miso in rats. *Hypertens Res*. V2006;29(9):731-8.

348 Ahymad IU, et al. Soy isoflavones in conjunction with radiation therapy in patients with prostate cancer. *Nutr Cancer*. 2010;62(7):996-1000.

349 Tacyildiz N, et al. Soy isoflavones ameliorate the adverse effects of chemotherapy in children. *Nutr Cancer*. 2010;62(7):1001-5.

350 Wu CH, Chou CC. Enhancement of aglycone, vitamin K2 and superoxide dismutase activity of black soybean through fermentation with Bacillus subtilis BCRC 14715 at different temperatures. *J Agric Food Chem*. 2009 Nov 25;57(22):10695-700.

351 Higashi-Okai K, et al. Potent antioxidative and antigenotoxic activity in aqueous extract of Japanese rice bran – association with peroxidase activity. *Phytother Res*. 2004 Aug;18(8):628-33.

352 Okai Y, Higashi-Okai K. Radical-scavenging activity of hot water extract of Japanese rice bran – association with phenolic acids. *J UOEH*. 2006 Mar 1;28(1):1-12.

353 Kativar SK. Green tea prevents non-melanoma skin cancer by enhancing DNA repair. *Arch Biochem Biophys*. 2011 Apr 15;508(2):152-8.

354 Liu ML, Wen JQ, Fan YB. Potential protection of green tea polyphenols against 1800 MHz electromagnetic radiation-induced Injury on rat cortical neurons. *Neurotox Res*. 2011 Oct;20(3):270-6.

355 Colloway DH, et al. Reduction of X-radiation mortality by cabbage and broccoli. *Proc Soc Exptl Biol Med*. 1959;100:405.

356 Colloway DH, et al. Further studies on reduction of X-radiation of Guinea Pigs by plant materials. *Quartermaster Food and Container Institute for the Armed Forces Report*. N.R. 1961:12-61.

357 Stoewsand GS. Bioactive organosulfur phytochemicals in Brassica oleracea vegetables – a review. *Food Chem Toxicol*. 1995 Jun;33(6):537-43.

358 Cope RB, Loehr C, Dashwood R, Kerkvliet NI.Ultraviolet radiation-induced non-melanoma skin cancer in the Crl:SKH1:hr-BR hairless mouse: augmentation of tumor multiplicity by chlorophyllin and protection by indole-3-carbinol. *Photochem Photobiol Sci*. 2006 May;5(5):499-507.

359 Suzuki K, et al. Relationship between serum carotenoids and hyperglycemia: A population-based cross-sectional study. *J Epidem*. 2002 Sep;12(5):357-64.

360 Aisa Y, et al. Fucoidan induces apoptosis of human HS-sultan cells accompanied by activation of caspase-3 and down-regulation of ERK pathways. *American Journal of Hematology*. 2005 Jan;78(1): 7–14.

361 Maruyama H, Yamamoto I. Suppression of 125I-uptake in mouse thyroid by seaweed feeding: possible preventative effect of dietary seaweed on internal radiation injury of the thyroid by radioactive iodine. *Kitasato Arch Exp Med*. 1992 Dec;65(4):209-16.

362 Gong YF, et al. Suppression of radioactive strontium absorption by sodium alginate in animals and human subjects. *Biomed Environ Sci*. 1991 Sep;4(3):273-82.

363 Hollriegl V, Rohmuss M, Oeh U, Roth P. Strontium biokinetics in humans: influence of alginate on the uptake of ingested strontium. *Health Phys*. 2004 Feb;86(2):193-6.

364 Maruyama H, Tamauchi H, Iizuka M, Nakano T. The role of NK cells in antitumor activity of dietary fucoidan from Undaria pinnatifida sporophylls (Mekabu). *Planta Med*. 2006 Dec;72(15):1415-7.

365 Suzuki K, et al. Relationship between serum carotenoids and hyperglycemia: a population-based cross-sectional study. *J Epidem*. 2002 Sep;12(5):357-64.

366 Shashkina MY, Shashkin PN, Sergeevi AV. Medicinal plants: chemical and medicobiological properties of chaga (Review). *Pharmaceutical Chemistry Journal*. 2006;40(10):560-8.

367 Wang DH, Weng XC. [Antitumor activity of extracts of Ganoderma lucidum and their protective effects on damaged HL-7702 cells induced by radiotherapy and chemotherapy]. *Zhongguo Zhong Yao Za Zhi*. 2006 Oct;31(19):1618-22.

368 Suzuki K, et al. Relationship between serum carotenoids and hyperglycemia: A population-based cross-sectional study. *J Epidem*. 2002 Sep;12(5):357-64.

369 Suzuki K, et al. Relationship between serum carotenoids and hyperglycemia: A population-based cross-sectional study. *J Epidem*. 2002 Sep;12(5):357-64.

370 See: http://www.japan-guide.com/e/e2347.html.

371 Higashi-Okai K, et al. Potent antioxidative and antigenotoxic activity in aqueous extract of Japanese rice bran – association with peroxidase activity. *Phytother Res*. 2004 Aug;18(8):628-33.

372 Suzuki M, Tanaka K, Kuwano M, Yoshida KT. Expression pattern of inositol phosphate-related enzymes in rice (Oryza sativa L.): implications for the phytic acid biosynthetic pathway. *Gene*. 2007 Dec 15;405(1-2):55-64.

373 Okai Y, Higashi-Okai K. Radical-scavenging activity of hot water extract of Japanese rice bran – association with phenolic acids. *J UOEH*. 2006 Mar 1;28(1):1-12.

374 Sorenson JR. Cu, Fe, Mn, and Zn chelates offer a medicinal chemistry approach to overcoming radiation injury. *Curr Med Chem*. 2002 Mar;9(6):639-62.

375 See: http://blogs.forbes.com/jeffmcmahon/2011/04/09/radiation-detected-in-drinking-water-in-13-more-us-cities-cesium-137-in-vermont-milk/.

376 Mehli H, Skuterud L, Mosdøl A, Tønnessen A. The impact of Chernobyl fallout on the Southern Saami reindeer herders of Norway in 1996. *Health Phys*. 2000 Dec;79(6):682-90.

377 Gastberger M, Steinhäusler F, Gerzabek MH, Hubmer A. Fallout strontium and caesium transfer from vegetation to cow milk at two lowland and two Alpine pastures. *J Environ Radioact*. 2001;54(2):267-73.

378 See: http://blogs.forbes.com/jeffmcmahon/2011/04/27/radioactive-strontium-found-in-hilo-hawaii-milk/.

379 See: http://www.epa.gov/radiation/docs/rert/radnet-cart-filter-final.pdf.

380 See: http://www.greenfacts.org/en/chernobyl/l-3/3-chernobyl-environment.htm.

381 See: http://www.heraldsun.com.au/news/hong-kong-finds-radioactive-iodine-in-fish/story-e6frf7jo-1226064532488.

382 See: http://www.nsf.gov/news/news_summ.jsp?cntn_id=119577&org=NSF&from=news.

383 See: http://www.greenpeace.org/international/en/news/Blogs/nuclear-reaction/marine-life-soaking-up-radiation-along-fukush/blog/34979.

384 See: http://www3.nhk.or.jp/daily/english/28_23.html.

385 China's State Oceanic Administration. Wider ocean contamination than Japanese government has admitted. *Asahi Shinbun* (12:08PM JST 8/16/2011). See: http://www.stdaily.com/kjrb/content/2011-08/15/content_337229.htm.

386 North Atlantic: Cod, Pollock, Blue Whiting and Red Hake; Haddock; Herring; Mackerel; Salmon; Tuna – Bluefin, Yellowfin and Longfin albacore; Yellowtail; Black Sea Bass; Monkfish (Angler Fish).

387 See: http://www.greenfacts.org/en/chernobyl/l-3/3-chernobyl-environment.htm.

388 Policy Issue Information, June 9th, 2011. SECY-11-0078. For: The Commissioners. From: R.W. Borchardt, Executive Director for Operations. Subject: U.S. Environmental Protection Agency Revisions To The Protective Action Guidance Manual; page 4. Contact: Patricia A. Milligan, NSIR/DPR. Telephone: 301-415-2223.

389 Maruyama H, Yamamoto I. Suppression of 125I-uptake in mouse thyroid by seaweed feeding: possible preventative effect of dietary seaweed on internal radiation injury of the thyroid by radioactive iodine. *Kitasato Arch Exp Med*. 1992 Dec;65(4):209-16.

390 Weiss JF, Landauer MR. History and development of radiation-protective agents. *Int J Radiat Biol*. 2009 Jul;85(7):539-73.

391 Gong YF, et al. Suppression of radioactive strontium absorption by sodium alginate in animals and human subjects. *Biomed Environ Sci*. 1991 Sep;4(3):273-82.

392 Hill P, Schläger M, Vogel V, Hille R, Nesterenko AV, Nesterenko VB. Studies on the current 137Cs body burden of children in Belarus – can the dose be further reduced? *Radiat Prot Dosimetry*. 2007;125(1-4):523-6.

393 Nesterenko VB, Nesterenko AV. Decorporation of Chernobyl radionuclides. *Ann N Y Acad Sci*. 2009 Nov;1181(1):303-10.

394 Maruyama H, Yamamoto I. Suppression of 125I-uptake in mouse thyroid by seaweed feeding: possible preventative effect of dietary seaweed on internal radiation injury of the thyroid by radioactive iodine. *Kitasato Arch Exp Med*. 1992 Dec;65(4):209-16.

395 See: http://www.optimox.com/pics/Iodine/pdfs/IOD01.pdf.

396 Nagataki S, Shizume K, Nakao K. Thyroid function in chronic excess iodide ingestion: Comparison of thyroidal absolute iodine uptake and degradation of thyroxine in euthyroid Japanese subjects. *J Clin Endo*. 1967;27:638-47.

397 United States National Research Council. *Dietary Reference Intakes for Vitamin A, Vitamin K, Arsenic, Boron, Chromium, Copper, Iodine, Iron, Manganese, Molybdenum, Nickel, Silicon, Vanadium, and Zinc*. National Academies Press. 2000;258–259.See: http://books.nap.edu/openbook.php?record_id=10026&page=258.

398 Abraham GE, Flechas JD, Hakala JC. Optimum levels of iodine for greatest mental and physical health. The *Original Internist*. 2000;9:5-20. See: http://www.optimox.com/pics/Iodine/IOD-01/IOD_01.htm.

399 Abraham GE, The Wolff-Chaikoff effect of increasing iodide intake on the thyroid. *Townsend Letter*. 2003;(245):100-1.

400 Abraham GE. The safe and effective implementation of orthoiodosupplementation in medical practice. The *Original Internist*. 2004 Apr;11:17-36. See: http://www.optimox.com/pics/Iodine/IOD-05/IOD_05.html.

401 Readers would do well to look for a physician who utilizes all types of healing systems as appropriate for the condition. In the early 1900s, physicians of this type were known as eclectic physicians. Today, eclectic physicians establish the context of the patient's illness or wellness according to their body constitution and do so

from the cellular level. Then, the physician integrates all forms of healing for the best patient outcome. Hormesis is routinely used by eclectic physicians when they incorporate homeopathic medicines at precise dilutions (potencies) into patient management. When incorporated properly, select potencies will induce the body's secretions of growth factors to enable rapid and complete healing, or target and accelerate specific toxins for elimination, which then leads the way to enable rapid and complete healing.

402 Abraham GE, Flechas JD. The effect of daily ingestion of 100mg iodine combined with high doses of Vitamins B2 and B3 (ATP cofactors) in five subjects with Fibromyalgia. *The Original Internist*. 2008 Mar;15(1):8-15. See: http://www.optimox.com/pics/Iodine/IOD-21/IOD_21.htm.

403 Brownstein D. *Iodine: Why You Need It, Why You Can't Live Without It*. 4th edition, Medical Alternative Press. W. Bloomfield, MI, 2009;97-124.

404 Abraham GE. Iodine supplementation markedly increases urinary excretion of fluoride and bromide. *Townsend Letter*. 2003;(238):108-9.

405 Abraham GE, Brownstein D. Evidence that the administration of Vitamin C improves a defective cellular transport mechanism for iodine: A case report. *The Original Internist*. 2005;12(3):125-30. See: http://www.optimox.com/pics/Iodine/IOD-11/IOD_11.htm.

406 Cline J. Effect of nutrient potassium on the intake of Cesium-137 and potassium on discrimination factor. *Nature*. 1962;193:1302-3.

407 Committee on Food Protection, Food and Nutrition Board, National Academy of Sciences. *Radionuclides in Foods*. National Academy Press. 1973:22-56.

408 Wasserman H, Comer C. Effect of dietary calcium and phosphorus levels on body burden of ingested radiostrontium. *Proc Soc Exp Biol Med*. 1960;103:124.

409 Palmer R, et al. Effect of calcium deposition on strontium-90 and calcium-45 in rats. *Science*. 1958;127:1505.

410 Apostoaei AI. Absorption of strontium from the gastrointestinal tract into plasma in healthy human adults. *Health Phys*. 2002 Jul;83(1):56-65.

411 Iyengar GV, et al. Dietary intakes of seven elements of importance in radiological protection by asian population: comparison with ICRP data. *Health Phys*. 2004 Jun;86(6):557-64.

412 Wagner AE, Ernst I, Iori R, Desel C, Rimbach G. Sulforaphane but not ascorbigen, indole-3-carbinole and ascorbic acid activates the transcription factor Nrf2 and induces phase-2 and antioxidant enzymes in human keratinocytes in culture. *Exp Dermatol*. 2010 Feb;19(2):137-44.

413 Wagner AE, et al. Ascorbic acid partly antagonizes resveratrol mediated heme oxygenase-1 but not paraoxonase-1 induction in cultured hepatocytes – role of the redox-regulated transcription factor Nrf2. *BMC Complement Altern Med*. 2011 Jan 3;11:1.

414 Okunieff P, et al. Antioxidants reduce consequences of radiation exposure. *Adv Exp Med Biol*. 2008;614:165-78.

415 Yamabe S, Kaneko K, Inoue H, Takita T. Maturation of fermented rice-koji miso can be monitored by an increase in fatty acid ethyl ester. *Biosci Biotechnol Biochem*. 2004 Jan;68(1):250-2.

416 Wattanathorn J, et al. Zingiber officinale mitigates brain damage and improves memory impairment in focal cerebral ischemic rat. *Evidence-Based Complementary and Alternative Medicine*. 2011;2011:Article ID 429505, Hindawi Publishing Corp.

417 Kabuto H, et al. Zingerone [4-(4-hydroxy-3-methoxyphenyl)-2-butanone] prevents 6-hydroxydopamine-induced dopamine depression in mouse striatum and increases superoxide scavenging activity in serum. *Neurochem Res*. 2005 Mar;30(3):325-32.

418 Wagner AE, Boesch-Saadatmandi C, Dose J, Schultheiss G, Rimbach G. Anti-inflammatory potential of allyl-isothiocyanate-role of Nrf2, NFκB and microRNA-155. *J Cell Mol Med*. 2011 Jun 22; doi: 10.1111/j.1582-4934.2011.01367.x. [Epub ahead of print].

419 Tsai PY, et al. Epigallocatechin-3-gallate prevents lupus nephritis development in mice via enhancing the Nrf2 antioxidant pathway and inhibiting NLRP3 inflammasome activation. *Free Radic Biol Med*. 2011 Aug 1;51(3):744-54.

420 Palsamy P, Subramanian S. Resveratrol protects diabetic kidney by attenuating hyperglycemia-mediated oxidative stress and renal inflammatory cytokines via Nrf2-Keap1 signaling. *Biochim Biophys Acta*. 2011 Jul;1812(7):719-31..

421 Preparing Miso soup to retain the maximal radio-protective effects requires a very precise method. First, boil vegetables in pure, uncontaminated water until the vegetables soften. Then, remove them from the heat. As the boiling pot cools down to ~150 degrees Fahrenheit (150oF), add dried seaweed so that it may reconstitute itself in the broth. After a few more minutes, add the Miso paste when the temperature approaches 140oF. Press the Miso paste into the still hot water with the back of a spoon. In this fashion, the raw food factors of: (A) the sun-dried seaweed plus (B) the fermentative bacteria of the Miso, plus (C) the heat sensitive Miso antioxidants (i.e., Genistein, isoflavones, saponins, etc....) are all properly preserved to perform their respective radioprotective roles.

422 Rate Limited – In this context, it means that supplies of essential or vital molecules that operate our antioxidant systems are critical to its continued optimal function in a crisis.

423 Michiels C, Raes M, Toussaint O, Remacle J. Importance of Se-glutathione peroxidase, catalase, and Cu/Zn-SOD for cell survival against oxidative stress. *Free Radic Biol Med*. 1994 Sep;17(3):235-48.

424 Giovannini C, et al. Polyphenols and endogenous antioxidant defences: effects on glutathione and glutathione related enzymes. *Ann Ist Super Sanita*. 2006;42(3):336-47.

425 Jones W, et al. Uptake, recycling, and antioxidant actions of alpha-lipoic acid in endothelial cells. *Free Radic Biol Med*. 2002 Jul 1;33(1):83-93.

426 Schecter SR. Fighting *Radiation with Foods, Herbs & Vitamins: Documented Natural Remedies That Boost Your Immunity and Detoxify*. East-West Health Books, Brookline, MA, 1992 Jan;pp.101-5.

427 Littarru GP, Tiano L. Bioenergetic and antioxidant properties of coenzyme Q10: recent developments. *Mol Biotechnol*. 2007 Sep;37(1):31-7.

428 Brown SL, et al. Antioxidant diet supplementation starting 24 hours after exposure reduces radiation lethality. *Radiat Res*. 2010 Apr;173(4):462-8.

429 Weiss JF, Landauer MR. Protection against ionizing radiation by antioxidant nutrients and phytochemicals. *Toxicology*. 2003 Jul 15;189(1-2):1-20.

430 Ambogenic means one nutrient (in this case selenium) can substitute for or be substituted by another nutrient (in this case Vitamin E).

431 Vitamin E becomes "spent" once it is oxidized. Once oxidized it loses its function as an antioxidant until recharged via reduction by Vitamin C or CoQ10(H).

432 Okunieff P, et al. Antioxidants reduce consequences of radiation exposure. *Adv Exp Med Biol*. 2008;614(168): 6.

433 Kaikkonen J, Tuomainen TP, Nyyssonen K, Salonen JT. Coenzyme Q10: absorption, antioxidative properties, determinants, and plasma levels. *Free Radic Res*. 2002 Apr;36(4):389-97.

434 Jones W, et al, Uptake, recycling, and antioxidant actions of alpha-lipoic acid in endothelial cells. *Free Radic Biol Med*. 2002 Jul 1;33(1):83-93.

435 May JM, Qu ZC, Neel DR, Li X. Recycling of Vitamin C from its oxidized forms by human endothelial cells. *Biochim Biophys Acta*. 2003 May 12;1640(2-3):153-61.

436 Calabrese V, Giuffrida Stella AM, Calvani M, Butterfield DA. Acetylcarnitine and cellular stress response: roles in nutritional redox homeostasis and regulation of longevity genes. *J Nutr Biochem*. 2006 Feb;17(2):73-88.

437 Calabrese V, et al. Redox homeostasis and cellular stress response in aging and neurodegeneration. *Methods Mol Biol*. 2010;610:285-308.

438 Neyfakh EA, Alimbekova AI, Ivanenko GF. Radiation-induced lipoperoxidative stress in children coupled with deficit of essential antioxidants. *Biochemistry* (Mosc). 1998 Aug;63(8):977-87.

439 Okunieff P, et al. Antioxidants reduce consequences of radiation exposure. *Adv Exp Med Biol*. 2008;614:165–78.

440 Nrf2 (NF-E2-Related Factor 2) – As a key human transcription factor, NrF2 regulates a cascade of select antioxidant and detoxifying genes involved in the production of S.O.D. and the glutathione family of antioxidant enzymes.

441 Karanjawala ZE, et al. Oxygen metabolism causes chromosome breaks and is associated with the neuronal apoptosis observed in DNA double-strand break repair mutants. *Curr Biol*. 2002 Mar 5;12(5):397-402.

442 Siu PM, et al. Habitual exercise increases resistance of lymphocytes to oxidant-induced DNA damage by upregulating expression of antioxidant and DNA repairing enzymes. *Exp Physiol*. 2011 Sep;96(9):889-906.

443 Szczesny B, Tann AW, Mitra S. Age and tissue-specific changes in mitochondrial and nuclear DNA base excision repair activity in mice: Susceptibility of skeletal muscles to oxidative injury. *Mech Ageing Dev.* 2010 May;131(5):330-7.

444 Kabuto et al. Zingerone [4-(4-hydroxy-3-methoxyphenyl)-2-butanone] prevents 6-hydroxydopamine-induced dopamine depression in mouse striatum and increases superoxide scavenging activity in serum. *Neurochem Res.* 2005;30(3):325-32.

445 Fouad AA, Al-Sultan AI, Refaie SM, Yacoubi MT. Coenzyme Q10 treatment ameliorates acute cisplatin nephrotoxicity in mice. *Toxicology.* 2010 Jul-Aug;274(1-3):49-56.

446 Demir EO, et al. N-acetyl-cysteine improves anastomotic wound healing after radiotherapy in rats. *J Invest Surg.* 2011;24(4):151-8.

447 Dani V, Dhawan D. Zinc as an antiperoxidative agent following iodine-131 induced changes on the antioxidant system and on the morphology of red blood cells in rats. *Hell J Nucl Med.* 2006 Jan-Apr;9(1):22-6.

448 Kaynar H. et al., Glutathione peroxidase, glutathione-S-transferase, catalase, xanthine oxidase, Cu-Zn superoxide dismutase activities, total glutathione, nitric oxide, and malondialdehyde levels in erythrocytes of patients with small cell and non-small cell lung cancer. *Cancer Lett.* 2005 Sep 28;227(2):133-9.

449 Amstad P, Moret R, Cerutti P. Glutathione peroxidase compensates for the hypersensitivity of Cu, Zn-superoxide dismutase overproducers to oxidant stress. *J Biol Chem.* 1994 Jan 21;269(3):1606-9.

450 Fouad AA, Al-Sultan AI, Refaie SM, Yacoubi MT. Coenzyme Q10 treatment ameliorates acute cisplatin nephrotoxicity in mice. *Toxicology.* 2010 Jul-Aug;274(1-3):49-56.

451 Olteanu H, Banerjee R. Human methionine synthase reductase, a soluble P-450 reductase-like dual flavoprotein, is sufficient for NADPH-dependent methionine synthase activation. *J Biol Chem.* 2001 Sep;276 (38): 35558–63.

452 Santos CX, et al. Redox signaling in cardiac myocytes. *Free Radic Biol Med.* 2011 Apr 1;50(7):777-93.

453 Zhao R, Masayasu H, Holmgren A. Ebselen: A substrate for human thioredoxin reductase strongly stimulating its hydroperoxide reductase activity and a superfast thioredoxin oxidant. *Proc Natl Acad Sci.* 2002 June 25; 99(13): 8579–84.

454 Calabrese V, et al. Redox regulation of cellular stress response in aging and neurodegenerative disorders: role of vitagenes. *Neurochem Res.* 2007 Apr-May;32(4-5):757-73.

455 Robbins MG, et al. Heat treatment of Brussels sprouts retains their ability to induce detoxification enzyme expression in vitro and in vivo. *J Food Sci.* 2011 Apr;76(3):C454-61.

456 Tanito M, et al. Sulforaphane induces thioredoxin through the antioxidant-responsive element and attenuates retinal light damage in mice. *Invest Ophthalmol Vis Sci.* 2005 Mar;46(3):979-87.

457 Zhao J, Yu S, Wu J, Lan L, Zhao Y. Curcumin and Nrf2 protect against neuronal oxidative stress and delayed death caused by oxygen and glucose deprivation. *Curr Neurovasc Res.* 2011 Jun 15.

458 ORAC = Oxygen radical absorbance (i.e., quenching) capacity.

459 See: http://articles.mercola.com/sites/articles/archive/2008/08/14/is-krill-oil-48-times-better-than-fish-oil.aspx.

460 See: http://www.neptunebiotech.com/images/documents/en/products/ORAC%20-%20Neptune%20Krill%20Oil%20Vs.%20Other%20oils%20ORAC.pdf.

461 Kidd PM. Omega-3 DHA and EPA for cognition, behavior, and mood: clinical findings and structural-functional synergies with cell membrane phospholipids. *Altern Med Rev.* 2007 Sep;12(3):207-27. See: http://krilloil.com/research-3.html.

462 See: http://products.mercola.com/astaxanthin/?source=nl.

463 Stocker R, et al. Ubiquinol-10 protects human low density lipoprotein more efficiently against lipid peroxidation than does alpha-tocopherol. *Proc Natl Acad Sci.* 1991;88:1646-50.

464 Bland J. *Clinical Breakthroughs in the Management of Chronic Fatigue Syndrome, Intestinal Dysbiosis, Immune Dysregulation and Cellular Toxicity*. HealthComm Inc., Gig Harbor, WA 1992;306.

465 Hultberg G, Andersson A, Isaksson A. Lipoic acid increases glutathione production and enhances the effect of mercury in human cell lines. *Toxicology*. 2002 Jun14;175(1-3):103-10.

466 Zhao R, Masayasu H, Holmgren A. Ebselen: A substrate for human thioredoxin reductase strongly stimulating its hydroperoxide reductase activity and a superfast thioredoxin oxidant. *Proc Natl Acad Sci*. 2002 June 25; 99(13): 8579–84.

467 Okunieff P, et al. Antioxidants reduce consequences of radiation exposure. *Adv Exp Med Biol*. 2008;614:167.

468 Brown SL, et al. Antioxidant diet supplementation starting 24 hours after exposure reduces radiation lethality. *Radiat Res*. 2010 Apr;173(4):462-8.

469 Atasoy BM, et al. Prophylactic feeding with immune-enhanced diet ameliorates chemoradiation-induced gastrointestinal injury in rats. *Int J Radiat Biol*. 2010 Oct;86(10):867-79.

470 Wambi CO, et al. Protective effects of dietary antioxidants on proton total-body irradiation-mediated hematopoietic cell and animal survival. *Radiat Res*. 2009 Aug;172(2):175-86.

471 Okunieff P, et al. Antioxidants reduce consequences of radiation exposure. *Adv Exp Med Biol*. 2008;614:165-6.

472 Mladenov E, Iliakis G. Induction and repair of DNA double strand breaks: the increasing spectrum of non-homologous end joining pathways. *Mutat Res*. 2011 Jun 3;711(1-2):61-72.

473 Frankenberg-Schwager M, The role of nonhomologous DNA end joining, conservative homologous recombination, and single-strand annealing in the cell cycle-dependent repair of DNA double-strand breaks induced by H(2)O(2) in mammalian cells. *Radiat Res*. 2008 Dec;170(6):784-93.

474 Bellés M, et al. Melatonin reduces uranium-induced nephrotoxicity in rats. *J Pineal Res*. 2007 Aug;43(1):87-95.

475 Shirazi A, Ghobadi G, Ghazi-Khansari M. A radiobiological review on melatonin: a novel radioprotector. *J Radiat Res* (Tokyo). 2007 Jul;48(4):263-72.

476 Reiter RJ, et al. Mechanisms for the protective actions of melatonin in the central nervous system. *Ann N Y Acad Sci*. 2001;939:200-15.

477 Reiter RJ, Acuña-Castroviejo D, Tan DX, Burkhardt S. Free radical-mediated molecular damage. Mechanisms for the protective actions of melatonin in the central nervous system. *Ann N Y Acad Sci*. 2001 Jun;939:200-15.

478 Negi G, Kumar A, Sharma SS. Melatonin modulates neuroinflammation and oxidative stress in experimental diabetic neuropathy: effects on NF-κB and Nrf2 cascades. *J Pineal Res*. 2011 Mar;50(2):124-31.

479 Srinivasan V, et al. Melatonin, immune function and aging. *Immunity & Ageing*. 2005;2:17.

480 Martin M, et al. Melatonin but not Vitamin C and E maintains glutathione homeostasis in t-butyl hydroperoxide-induced mitochondrial oxidative stress. *FASEB J*. 2000;14:1677-9.

481 Okunieff P, et al. Antioxidants reduce consequences of radiation exposure. *Adv Exp Med Biol*. 2008;614:3 (or p.168 in original journal).

482 Undeger U, Giray B, Zorlu AF, Oge K, Baçaran N. Protective effects of melatonin on the ionizing radiation induced DNA damage in the rat brain. *Exp Toxicol Pathol*. 2004 Mar;55(5):379-84.

483 Vijayalaxmi et al. Melatonin as a radioprotective agent: a review. *Int J Radiat Oncol Biol Phys*. 2004 Jul1;59(3):639-53.

484 Valko M, et al. Free radicals, metals and antioxidants in oxidative stress-induced cancer. *Chem Biol Interact*. 2006 Mar 10;160(1):1-40.

485 Varnes ME, Biaglow JE, Roizin-Towle L, Hall EJ. Depletion of intracellular GSH and NPSH by buthionine sulfoximine and diethyl maleate: factors that influence enhancement of aerobic radiation response. *Int J Radiat Oncol Biol Phys*. 1984 Aug;10(8):1229-33.

486 Biaglow JE, Varnes ME, Clark EP, Epp ER. The role of thiols in cellular response to radiation and drugs. *Radiat Res*. 1983 Sep;95(3):437-55.

487 Chung SW, et al. Molecular delineation of gamma-Ray-Induced NF-kappaB activation and pro-inflammatory genes in SMP30 knockout mice. *Radiat Res*. 2010 May;173(5):629-34.

488 Brown SL, et al. Antioxidant diet supplementation starting 24 hours after exposure reduces radiation lethality. *Radiat Res*. 2010 Apr;173(4):462-8.

489 Tak JK, Park JW. The use of ebselen for radioprotection in cultured cells and mice. *Free Radic Biol Med*. 2009 Apr 15;46(8):1177-85.

490 Wambi CO, et al. Protective effects of dietary antioxidants on proton total-body irradiation-mediated hematopoietic cell and animal survival. *Radiat Res*. 2009 Aug;172(2):175-86.

491 Breccia A, et al. Chemical radioprotection by organic selenium compounds in vivo. *Radiat Res* (University of Bologna), 1969 Jun;38:483-92.

492 Franca CA, et al. Serum levels of selenium in patients with breast cancer before and after treatment of external beam radiotherapy. *Ann Oncol*. 2011 May;22(5):1109-12.

493 Brown SL, et al. Antioxidant diet supplementation starting 24 hours after exposure reduces radiation lethality. *Radiat Res*. 2010 Apr;173(4):462-8.

494 Tuji FM, et al. Ultrastructural assessment of the radioprotective effects of sodium selenite on parotid glands in rats. *J Oral Sci*. 2010;52(3):369-75.

495 Zhao W, Goswami PC, Robbins ME. Radiation-induced up-regulation of Mmp2 involves increased mRNA stability, redox modulation, and MAPK activation. *Radiat Res*. 2004 Apr;161(4):418-29.

496 Bland J. *Clinical Breakthroughs in the Management of: Chronic Fatigue Syndrome, Intestinal Dysbiosis, Immune Dysregulation and Cellular Toxicity*. HealthComm Inc., Gig Harbor, WA 1992.

497 Okunieff P, et al. Antioxidants reduce consequences of radiation exposure. *Adv Exp Med Biol*. 2008;614:168.

498 Bishayee A, et al. Resveratrol suppresses oxidative stress and inflammatory response in diethylnitrosamine-initiated rat hepatocarcinogenesis. *Cancer Prev Res* (Phila Pa). 2010 Jun;3(6):753-63.

499 Ping Z, et al. Sulforaphane protects brains against hypoxic-ischemic injury through induction of Nrf2-dependent phase 2 enzyme. *Brain Res*. 2010 Apr 24.

500 Romeo L. et al. The major green tea polyphenol, (-)-epigallocatechin-3-gallate, induces heme oxygenase in rat neurons and acts as an effective neuroprotective agent against oxidative stress. *J Am Coll Nutr*. 2009 Aug;28 Suppl:492S-9S.

501 Yang C, et al. Curcumin upregulates transcription factor Nrf2, HO-1 expression and protects rat brains against focal ischemia. *Brain Res*. 2009 Jul 28;1282:133-41.

502 Romanque P, Cornejo P, Valdés S, Videla LA. Thyroid hormone administration induces rat liver nrf2 activation: suppression by N-acetylcysteine pretreatment. *Thyroid*. 2011 Jun;21(6):655-62.

503 See: http://www.epa.gov/japan2011/rert/radnet-sampling-data.html

504 Hindle AA, Hall EA. Dipicolinic acid (DPA) assay revisited and appraised for spore detection. *Analyst*. 1999 Nov;124(11):1599-604.

505 Kort R, et al. Assessment of heat resistance of bacterial spores from food product isolates by fluorescence monitoring of dipicolinic Acid Release. *Appl Environ Microbiol*. 2005 July;71(7): 3556–64.

506 Soil radionuclide transfer ➔ to plant attests to cabbage's powers of radionuclide "chelation." When ingested, isothiocyanates, indoles (I3C) and sulforaphane

content of the cabbage family are known to aid elimination of toxic metals and other xenobiotics. One known mechanism involves their conjugation to bodily stores of NAC; another with the increased production of glutathione via Nrf2 upregulation. The latter two are well known chelators to radionuclides.

507 Ban-Nai T, Muramatsu Y, Yanagisawa K. Transfer factors of some selected radionuclides (radioactive Cs, Sr, Mn, Co and Zn) from soil to leaf vegetables. *J Radiat Res* (Tokyo). 1995 Jun;36(2):143-54.

508 Paasikallio A, Rantavaara A, Sippola J. The transfer of cesium-137 and strontium-90 from soil to food crops after the Chernobyl accident. *Sci Total Environ*. 1994 Oct 14;155(2):109-24.

509 Unsworth EF, et al. Investigations of the use of clay minerals and prussian blue in reducing the transfer of dietary radiocaesium to milk. *Sci Total Environ*. 1989 Sep;85:339-47.

510 Brynildsen LI, Selnaes TD, Strand P, Hove K. Countermeasures for radiocesium in animal products in Norway after the Chernobyl accident – techniques, effectiveness, and costs. *Health Phys*. 1996 May;70(5):665-72.

511 Unsworth EF, et al. Investigations of the use of clay minerals and prussian blue in reducing the transfer of dietary radiocaesium to milk. *Sci Total Environ*. 1989 Sep;85:339-47.

512 Nesterenko VB, Nesterenko AV, Babenko VI, Yerkovich TV,Babenko IV. Reducing the 137Cs-load in the organism of "Chernobyl" children with apple-pectin. *Swiss Med Wkly*. 2004;134:24-7.

513 Hill P, et al. Studies on the current 137Cs body burden of children in Belarus – can the dose be further reduced? *Radiat Prot Dosimetry*. 2007;125(1-4):523-6.

514 Bandazhevskaya GS, Nesterenko VB, Babenko VI, Yerkovich TV, Bandazhevsky YI. Relationship between caesium (137Cs) load, cardiovascular symptoms, and source of food in 'Chernobyl' children – preliminary observations after intake of oral apple pectin. *Swiss Med Wkly*. 2004 Dec 18;134(49-50):725-9.

515 Chaitow L, Trenev N. *Probiotics.* Thorsons, Hammersmith, London, 1990:118-20, & 144.

516 Blom H, Mortvedt T. Anti-microbial substances produced by food associated micro-organisms. *Biochem Soc Trans Food Biotech*. 1991;694-8.

517 Jagtap VS, et al. An effective and better strategy for reducing body burden of radiostrontium. *J Radiol Prot*. 2003 Sep;23(3):317-26.

518 Hollriegl V, Rohmuss M, Oeh U, Roth P. Strontium biokinetics in humans: influence of alginate on the uptake of ingested strontium. *Health Phys*. 2004 Feb;86(2):193-6.

519 Gong YF, et al. Suppression of radioactive strontium absorption by sodium alginate in animals and human subjects. *Biomed Environ Sci*. 1991 Sep;4(3):273-82.

520 Some distinguishable properties between acid-stable and neutral types of alpha-amylases from acid-producing koji. *J Biosci Bioeng*. 2007 Nov;104(5):353-62.

521 Ertan F, Yagar H, Balkan B. Optimization of alpha-amylase immobilization in calcium alginate beads. *Prep Biochem Biotechnol*. 2007;37(3):195-204.

522 Kubrak OI, Lushchak VI. Optimization of conditions for immobilization of alpha-amylase from Bacillus sp. BKL20 in Ca2+-alginate beads. *Ukr Biokhim Zh*. 2008 Nov-Dec;80(6):32-41.

523 Tanaka Y, et al. Studies on the inhibition of intestinal absorption of radioactive strontium VL alginate degradation products as potent in vivo. *Canad Med Ass J*. 1968 Jun 22 & 29;98:1180.

524 Horikoshi T, et al. Uptake of Uranium by various cell fractions of chlorella regularis. *Radioisotopes*. 1979 Aug;28(8):485-7.

525 Flowers JL, et al. Clinical evidence supporting the use of an activated clinoptilolite suspension as an agent to increase urinary excretion of toxic heavy metals. *Nutrition and Dietary Supplements*. 2009:1 11–18.

526 Chapman KW, Chupas PJ, Nenoff TM. Radioactive iodine capture in silver-containing mordenites through nanoscale silver iodide formation. *J Am Chem Soc*. 2010 Jul 7;132(26):8897-9.

527 Dyer A, Las T, Zubair M. The use of natural zeolites for radioactive waste treatment: studies on leaching from zeolite/cement composites. *Journal of Radioanalytical and Nuclear Chemistry*. 2000;243(3):839-41.

528 Forberg S, Jones B, Westermark T. Can zeolites decrease the uptake and accelerate the excretion of radio-caesium in ruminants? *Sci Total Environ*. 1989;79:37–41.

529 Zhang GH, Liu XS, Thomas JK. Radiation induced physical and chemical processes in zeolite materials. *Radiation Physics And Chemistry*. 1998 Feb;51(2):135-52.

530 Goto K. A study of the acidosis, blood urea, and plasma chlorides in uranium nephritis in the dog, and of the protective action of sodium bicarbonate. *JEM*. 1917;25(5):693-719.

531 Destombes C, Laroche P, Cazoulat A, Gérasimo P. Reduction of renal uranium uptake by acetazolamide: the importance of urinary elimination of bicarbonate. *Ann Pharm Fr*. 1999 Sep;57(5):397-400.

532 Bellés M, et al. Melatonin reduces uranium-induced nephrotoxicity in rats. *J Pineal Res*. 2007 Aug;43(1):87-95.

533 Vijayalaxmi, Reiter RJ, Tan DX, Herman TS, Thomas CR Jr. Melatonin as a radioprotective agent: a review. *Int J Radiat Oncol Biol Phys*. 2004 Jul 1;59(3):639-53.

534 Wambi CO, et al. Protective effects of dietary antioxidants on proton total-body irradiation-mediated hematopoietic cell and animal survival. *Radiat Res*. 2009 Aug;172(2):175-86.

535 Reiter RJ, et al. Mechanisms for the Protective Actions of Melatonin in the Central Nervous System. *Ann N Y Acad Sci*. 2001;939:200-15.

536 Brown SL, et al. Antioxidant diet supplementation starting 24 hours after exposure reduces radiation lethality. *Radiat Res*. 2010 Apr;173(4):462-8.

537 Sorenson JR. Cu, Fe, Mn, and Zn chelates offer a medicinal chemistry approach to overcoming radiation injury. *Curr Med Chem*. 2002 Mar;9(6):639-62.

538 Taha EA, Hassan NY, Aal FA, Fattah Lel-S. Fluorimetric determination of some sulfur containing compounds through complex formation with terbium (Tb+3) and uranium (U+3). *J Fluoresc.* 2007 May; 17 (3):293-300.

539 Milgram S, Carrière M, Thiebault C, Malaval L, Gouget B. Cytotoxic and phenotypic effects of uranium and lead on osteoblastic cells are highly dependent on metal speciation. *Toxicology.* 2008 Aug 19; 250 (1):62-9.

540 Levitskaia TG, et al. Aminothiol receptors for decorporation of intravenously administered (60)Co in the rat. *Health Phys.* 2010 Jan;98(1):53-60.

541 Henge-Napoli MHEfficacy of 3,4,3-LIHOPO for reducing the retention of uranium in rat after acute administration. *Int J Radiat Biol.* 1995 Oct;68(4):389-93.

542 Henge-Napoli MH, et al. Efficacy of 3,4,3-LIHOPO for reducing the retention of uranium in rat after acute administration. *Int J Radiat Biol.* 1995 Oct;68(4):389-93.

543 Lin KA, Chen JH, Lee DF, Lin LY. Alkaline induces metallothionein gene expression and potentiates cell proliferation in Chinese hamster ovary cells. *J Cell Physiol.* 2005 Dec;205(3):428-36.

544 Fatome M. [Management of accidental internal exposure]. *J Radiol.* 1994 Nov;75(11):571-5

545 Fukuda S, et al. The effects of bicarbonate and its combination with chelating agents used for the removal of depleted uranium in rats. *Hemoglobin.* 2008;32(1-2):191-8.

546 *Dorland's Pocket Medical Dictionary.* Twenty-Third Edition, p.590.

547 *Webster's Ninth New Collegiate Dictionary*; p.991.

548 Wing S, et al. A case control study of multiple myeloma at four nuclear facilities. *Annals of Epidemiology.* 2000 Apr;10(3):144-53.

549 Ling GN. *Life at the Cell and Below-Cell Level: The Hidden History of a Fundamental Revolution in Biology.* Pacific Press, NY, 2001. See: www.gilbertling.org

550 Guyton AC. *Textbook of Medical Physiology.* Fifth Edition, WB Saunders Co., Philadelphia, PA, 1976, p. 12.

551 O'Connor A, et al., DNA double strand breaks in epidermal cells cause immune suppression in vivo and cytokine production in vitro. *J Immunol.* 1996;157(1):271-8.

552 Holz O, et al. Reproducibility of basal and induced DNA single-strand breaks detected by the single-cell gel electrophoresis assay in human peripheral mononuclear leukocytes. *Int Arch Occup Environ Health.* 1995;67(5):305-10.

553 Krause T, et al. A novel technique for the detection of DNA single-strand breaks in human white blood cells and its combination with the unscheduled DNA synthesis assay. *Assay Int Arch Occup Environ Health.* 1993;65(2):77-82.

554 Vojdani A, Ghoneum M, Choppa P. Minimizing cancer risk using molecular techniques: a review. *Toxicol Ind Health.* 1997;13(5):589-626.

555 Ling GN. *Life at the Cell and Below-Cell Level: The Hidden History of a Fundamental Revolution in Biology.* Pacific Press, NY, 2001;pp. 74-114; 154-232.

556 See: http://doctorapsley.com/FourPillars.aspx.

557 To live to at least 90 years of age, largely free of chronic illness.

558 Pende N. *Constitutional Inadequacies: An Introduction to the Study of Abnormal Constitutions*. Translated by Sante Nacearati, MD, PhD, Sc.D., published by Lea & Febriger, Philadelphia, PA, 1928.

559 Weston Price. *Nutrition and Physical Degeneration*. Price Pottenger Foundation (Editor). Price Pottenger Nutrition. 8th Edition. 2008.

560 Benet S. Abkhasians: *The Long-Living People of the Caucasus*. Holt, Rinehart and Winston, Inc., NY, 1974.

561 Pitskhelauri GZ. *The Long-Living of Soviet Georgia*. Human Sciences Press, 1982 Feb.

562 Buettner D. The blue zones: lessons for living longer from the people who've lived the longest. *National Geographic*, Washington D.C. 2008.

563 For full documentation, refer to*: The Regeneration Effect*: Volumes 1 – 6 due out in 2012. See: http://doctorapsley.com/EBooks.aspx.

564 Azzam EI, Raaphorst GP, Mitchel REJ. Radiation-induced adaptive response for cells. *Radiation Research*. 1994;138(1):S28-S31.

565 Kuwahara Y, et al. Enhancement of autophagy is a potential modality for tumors refractory to radiotherapy. *Cell Death Dis*. 2011 Jun 30;2:e177.

566 Chaachousay H, et al. Autophagy contributes to resistance of tumor cells to ionizing radiation. *Radiother Oncol*. 2011 Jun;99(3):287-92.

567 Behrends C, Sowa ME, Gygi SP, Harper JW. Network organization of the human autophagy system. *Nature*. 2010 Jul 1;466(7302):68-76.

568 Rayala SK, et al. Hepatocyte growth factor–regulated tyrosine kinase substrate (HRS) interacts with PELP1 and activates MAPK. *J Biol Chem*. 2006; 281:4395- 403.

569 The fresh juices of organic raw foods grown in mineral rich soils, and high quality whey are high-end sources of these.

570 Cope FW. Pathology of structured water and associated cations in cells (the tissue damage syndrome) and its medical treatment. *Physiol Chem Phys*. 1977;9(6):547-53.

571 Cope FW. Successful therapy of heart disease by high potassium together with low sodium in accord with predictions from the associated cation, structured water concept of the cell. *Physiol Chem Phys*. 1979;11(1):93-4.

572 Carra S, Seguin SJ, Landry J. HspB8 and Bag3: a new chaperone complex targeting misfolded proteins to macroautophagy. *Autophagy*. 2008 Feb;4(2):237-9.

573 Martinez-Outschoorn UE, et al. The autophagic tumor stroma model of cancer or "battery-operated tumor growth:" A simple solution to the autophagy paradox. *Cell Cycle*. 2010 Nov 1; 9:21, 4297-306.

574 During fasting or prolonged low calories diets, the body must use its own reserves of fat to fuel its essential metabolic needs. Fat must be broken down into ketone

bodies for this purpose, via a process known as Beta oxidation. Beta oxidation is dependent upon iodine.

575 Nakamura Y, et al. A combination of indol-3-carbinol and genistein synergistically induces apoptosis in human colon cancer HT-29 cells by inhibiting Akt phosphorylation and progression of autophagy. *Mol Cancer*. 2009 Nov 12;8:100.

576 Finn PF, Dice JF. Ketone bodies stimulate chaperone-mediated autophagy. *JBC*. 2005 Jul 8;280(27):25864-70.

577 Singletary K, Milner J. Diet, Autophagy, and Cancer: A Review. *Cancer Epidemiol Biomarkers Prev*. 2008 Jul;17(7):1596-610.

578 Mi L, Gan N, Fung-Lung Chung. Aggresome-like structure induced by isothiocyanates is novel proteasomes-dependent degradation machinery. *Biochem Biophys Res Commun*. 2009 Oct 16;388(2):456-62.

579 Li W, et al. EGCG stimulates autophagy and reduces cytoplasmic HMGB1 levels in endotoxin-stimulated macrophages. *Biochem Pharmacol*. 2011 May 1;81(9):1152-63.

580 Cohen HY, et al. Calorie restriction promotes mammalian cell survival by inducing the SIRT1 deacetylase. *Science*. 2004 Jul;305(5682):390–2.

581 Wu S, Sun J. Vitamin D, Vitamin D receptor, and macroautophagy in inflammation and infection. *Discov Med*. 2011 Apr;11(59):325-35.

582 Chen T, et al. Rapamycin and other longevity-promoting compounds enhance the generation of mouse induced pluripotent stem cells. *Aging Cell*. 2011 May 25. doi: 10.1111/j.1474-9726.2011.00722.x. [Epub ahead of print]

583 Fujita S, et al. Effect of Waon therapy on oxidative stress in chronic heart failure. *Circ J*. 2011 Feb;75(2):348-56.

584 Ohshiro K, Rayala SK, El-Naggar AK, Kumar R. Delivery of cytoplasmic proteins to autophagosomes. *Autophagy*. 2008 Jan;4(1):104-6.

585 Flavin DF. Reversing splenomegalies in Epstein Barr Virus infected children: mechanisms of toxicity in viral diseases. *JOM*. 2006 Second quarter;21(2):95-101.

586 Flavin, DF. Clinical patient studies: a lipoxygenase inhibitor in breast cancer brain metastases. *Journal of Neuro-Oncology.* 2007 Mar;82(1):91-3.

587 Sorenson JR. Cu, Fe, Mn, and Zn chelates offer a medicinal chemistry approach to overcoming radiation injury. *Curr Med Chem*. 2002 Mar;9(6):639-62.

588 Aravindan N, et al. Curcumin regulates low-linear energy transfer γ-radiation-induced NFκB-dependent telomerase activity in human neuroblastoma cells. *Int J Radiat Oncol Biol Phys*. 2011 Mar 15;79(4):1206-15.

589 Rafiee P, et al. Modulatory effect of curcumin on survival of irradiated human intestinal microvascular endothelial cells: role of Akt/mTOR and NF-{kappa}B. *Am J Physiol Gastrointest Liver Physiol*. 2010 Jun;298(6):G865-77.

590 Chittezhath M, Kuttan G. Radioprotective activity of naturally occurring organosulfur compounds. *Tumori*. 2006 Mar-Apr;92(2):163-9.

591 Zhang Y. Allyl isothiocyanate as a cancer chemopreventive phytochemical. *Mol Nutr Food Res*. 2010 Jan;54(1):127-35.

592 See: http://doctorapsley.com/AspirinandSynergistsforCancer.aspx.

593 Karanjawala ZE, et al. Oxygen metabolism causes chromosome breaks and is associated with the neuronal apoptosis observed in DNA double-strand break repair mutants. *Curr Biol*. 2002 Mar 5;12(5):397-402.

594 Siu PM, et al. Habitual exercise increases resistance of lymphocytes to oxidant-induced DNA damage by upregulating expression of antioxidant and DNA repairing enzymes. *Exp Physiol*. 2011 Sep;96(9):889-906.

595 Szczesny B, Tann AW, Mitra S. Age- and tissue-specific changes in mitochondrial and nuclear DNA base excision repair activity in mice: Susceptibility of skeletal muscles to oxidative injury. *Mech Ageing Dev*. 2010 May;131(5):330-7.

596 Barbe P, et al. Triiodothyronine-mediated up-regulation of UCP2 and UCP3 mRNA expression in human skeletal muscle without coordinated induction of mitochondrial respiratory chain genes. *FASEB J*. 2001 Jan;15(1):13-15.

597 Crunkhorn S, Patti ME. Links between thyroid hormone action, oxidative metabolism, and diabetes risk? *Thyroid*. 2008 Feb;18(2):227-37.

598 Carreau A, Hafny-Rahbi BE, Matejuk A, Grillon C, Kieda C. Why is the partial oxygen pressure of human tissues a crucial parameter? Small molecules and hypoxia. *J Cell Mol Med*. 2011 Jun;15(6):1239-53.

599 Watson G. *Nutrition and Your Mind: The Psychochemical Response*. Bantam Books, 1973.

600 von Ardenne M. *Oxygen Multistep Therapy: Physiological and Technical Foundations*. Translated by Paula Kirby & Winfred Kruger, Thieme, NY, 1990. www.thieme.com.

601 McNaughton LR, Siegler J, Midgley A. Ergogenic effects of sodium bicarbonate. *Curr Sports Med Rep*. 2008 Jul-Aug;7(4):230-6.

602 von Ardenne M. *Oxygen Multistep Therapy: Physiological and Technical Foundations*. Thieme, New York, 1990;p. 64-93.

603 Rwigema JC, et al. Two strategies for the development of mitochondrion-targeted small molecule radiation damage mitigators. *Int J Radiat Oncol Biol Phys*. 2011 Jul 1;80(3):860-8.

604 Rajendran S, Harrison SH, Thomas RA, Tucker JD. The role of mitochondria in the radiation-induced bystander effect in human lymphoblastoid cells. *Radiat Res*. 2011 Feb;175(2):159-71.

605 Leone et al. PGC-1alpha deficiency causes multi-system energy metabolic derangements: muscle dysfunction, abnormal weight control and hepatic steatosis. *PLoS Biol*. 2005;3(4): e101.

606 Ma YS, Wu SB, Lee WY, Cheng JS, Wei YH. Response to the increase of oxidative stress and mutation of mitochondrial DNA in aging. *Biochim Biophys Acta*. 2009 Oct;1790(10):1021-9.

607 Wei YH, Wu SB, Ma YS, Lee HC. Respiratory function decline and DNA mutation in mitochondria, oxidative stress and altered gene expression during aging. *Chang Gung Med J*. 2009 Mar-Apr;32(2):113-32.

608 Safdar A, et al. Exercise increases mitochondrial PGC-1alpha content and promotes nuclear-mitochondrial cross-talk to coordinate mitochondrial biogenesis. *J Biol Chem*. 2011 Mar 25;286(12):10605-17.

609 Ranhotra HS. Long-term caloric restriction up-regulates PPAR gamma co-activator 1 alpha (PGC-1alpha) expression in mice. *Indian J Biochem Biophys*. 2010 Oct;47(5):272-7.

610 PGC-1 α – Peroxisome proliferator-activated receptor-γ coactivator 1 α.

611 Lopez-Lluch G, et al. Mitochondrial biogenesis and healthy aging. *Exp Gerontol*. 2008;43(9):813.

612 Shoag J, Arany Z. Regulation of hypoxia-inducible genes by PGC-1 alpha. *Arterioscler Thromb Vasc Biol*. 2010 Apr;30(4):662-6.

613 Lanza IR et al. Endurance exercise as a countermeasure for aging. *Diabetes*. 2008;57(11):2933.

614 Nitric oxide (NO) is an extremely important gas produced in the body which facilitates cell signaling and vital cell-to-cell information flow.

615 Sirt1 (the enzyme sirtuin-1, also known as NAD+ dependent deacetylase) is another antioxidant enzyme that has significant influence over: (a) proper cell division, (b) proper fat metabolism, (c) preventing premature cell aging, and (d) proper apoptosis (programmed cell death).

616 AMPK (5' adenosine monophosphate-activated protein kinase) is a major player assuring proper cellular energy production and balance (homeostasis).

617 Knott AB, Bossy-Wetzel E. Impact of nitric oxide on metabolism in health and age-related disease. *Diabetes Obes Metab*. 2010 Oct;12 Suppl 2:126-33

618 Baluchnejadmojarad T, Roghani M. Chronic epigallocatechin-3-gallate ameliorates learning and memory deficits in diabetic rats via modulation of nitric oxide and oxidative stress. *Behav Brain Res*. 2011 Oct 31;224(2):305-10.

619 Vetterli L, Maechler P. Resveratrol-activated SIRT1 in liver and pancreatic β-cells: a Janus head looking to the same direction of metabolic homeostasis. *Aging* (Albany NY). 2011 Apr;3(4):444-9.

620 Packer L, Cadenas E. Lipoic acid: energy metabolism and redox regulation of transcription and cell signaling. *J Clin Biochem Nutr*. 2011 Jan;48(1):26-32.

621 Irrcher I, Adhihetty PJ, Sheehan T, Joseph AM, Hood DA. PPARgamma coactivator-1alpha expression during thyroid hormone- and contractile activity-induced mitochondrial adaptations. *Am J Physiol Cell Physiol*. 2003 Jun;284(6):C1669-77.

622 Hultberg G, Andersson A, Isaksson A. Lipoic acid increases glutathione production and enhances the effect of mercury in human cell lines. *Toxicology*. 2002 Jun14;175(1-3):103-10.

623 McCarty MF. Practical prevention of cardiac remodeling and atrial fibrillation with full-spectrum antioxidant therapy and ancillary strategies. *Med Hypotheses*. 2010 Aug;75(2):141-7.

624 Okello E, Jiang X, Mohamed S, Zhao Q, Wang T. Combined statin/coenzyme Q10 as adjunctive treatment of chronic heart failure. *Med Hypotheses*. 2009 Sep;73(3):306-8.

625 Chuang YC. Contribution of nitric oxide, superoxide anion, and peroxynitrite to activation of mitochondrial apoptotic signaling in hippocampal CA3 subfield following experimental temporal lobe status epilepticus. *Epilepsia*. 2009 Apr;50(4):731-46.

626 Deichmann R, Lavie C, Andrews S. Coenzyme q10 and statin-induced mitochondrial dysfunction. *Ochsner J*. 2010 Spring;10(1):16-21.

627 Delwing D, et al. Protective effect of antioxidants on cerebrum oxidative damage caused by arginine on pyruvate kinase activity. *Metab Brain Dis*. 2009 Sep;24(3):469-79.

628 Singer RB. Long-term comparative cancer mortality after use of radio-iodine in the treatment of hyperthyroidism, a fully reported multicenter study. *J Insur Med*. 2001;33(2):138-42.

629 Metso S, et al. Increased cardiovascular and cancer mortality after radioiodine treatment for hyperthyroidism. *J Clin Endocrinol Metab*. 2007 Jun;92(6):2190-6.

630 Metso S, et al. Increased long-term cardiovascular morbidity among patients treated with radioactive iodine for hyperthyroidism. *Clin Endocrinol* (Oxf). 2008 Mar;68(3):450-7.

631 Sawka AM, et al. Second primary malignancy risk after radioactive iodine treatment for thyroid cancer: a systematic review and meta-analysis. *Thyroid*. 2009 May;19(5):451-7.

632 Acharya SH, et al. Radioiodine therapy (RAI) for Graves' disease (GD) and the effect on ophthalmopathy: a systematic review. *Clin Endocrinol* (Oxf). 2008 Dec;69(6):943-50.

633 Metso S, et al. Increased cancer incidence after radioiodine treatment for hyperthyroidism. *Cancer*. 2007 May 15;109(10):1972-9.

634 Irrcher I, Adhihetty PJ, Sheehan T, Joseph AM, Hood DA. PPARgamma coactivator-1alpha expression during thyroid hormone- and contractile activity-induced mitochondrial adaptations. *Am J Physiol Cell Physiol.* 2003 Jun;284(6):C1669-77.

635 Starr M. *Hypothyroidism Type 2: The Epidemic*. Mark Starr Trust, Columbia, MO, 2007.

636 See: http://doctorapsley.com/Hypothyroidism.aspx.

637 Asami DK, Hong YJ, Barrett DM, Mitchell AE. Comparison of the total phenolic and ascorbic acid content of freeze-dried and air-dried marionberry, strawberry, and corn grown using conventional, organic, and sustainable agricultural practices. *J Agric Food Chem*. 2003 Feb 26;51(5):1237-41.

638 Davis DR. Declining fruit and vegetable nutrient composition: What is the evidence? *HortScience*. 2009 Feb;44(1):15-9.

639 United Nations Conference on Environments and Development (UNCED), Earth Summit, Rio de Janeiro, Brazil, June 3-14, 1992.

640 Lopez-Berenguer C, et al. Effects of microwave cooking conditions on bioactive compounds present in broccoli inflorescences. *J Agric Food Chem*. 2007 Nov 28;55(24):10001-7.

641 Hemalatha S, Platel K, Srinivasan K. Influence of heat processing on the bioaccessibility of zinc and iron from cereals and pulses consumed in India. *J Trace Elem Med Biol*. 2007;21(1):1-17.

642 Elizalde-Gonzalez MP, Hernandez-Ogarcia SG. Effect of cooking process on the contents of two bioactive carotenoids in Solanum lycopersicum tomatoes and Physalis ixocarpa and Physalis philadelphica tomatillos. *Molecules.* 2007 Aug13;12(8):1829-35.

643 Fisher A. Nature of the growth-accelerating substances of animal tissue cells. *Nature*. 1939;144:113.

644 Cope FW. Pathology of structured water and associated cations in cells (the tissue damage syndrome) and its medical treatment. *Physiol Chem Phys*. 1977;9(6):547-53.

645 Phillips PA, et al. Reduced thirst after water deprivation in healthy elderly men. *NEJM*. 1984 Sep 20;311(12):753-9.

646 Cope FW. Successful therapy of heart disease by high potassium together with low sodium in accord with predictions from the associated cation, structured water concept of the cell. *Physiol Chem Phys*. 1979;11(1):93-4.

647 Lourau M, Lartigue O. The influence of diet on the biological effects produced by whole body irradiation. *Experientia*. 1950;6:25.

648 Guo S, et al. Protective activity of different concentration of tea polyphenols and its major compound EGCG against whole body irradiation-induced injury in mice. *Zhongguo Zhong Yao Za Zhi*. 2010 May;35(10):1328-31.

649 Behrends C, Sowa ME, Gygi SP, Harper JW. Network organization of the human autophagy system. *Nature*. 2010 July 1; 466(7302): 68–76.

650 Rodriguez-Rocha H, Garcia-Garcia A, Panayiotidis MI, Franco R. DNA damage and autophagy. *Mutat Res*. 2011 Jun 3;711(1-2):158-66.

651 Croteau DL, Peng Y, Van Houten B. DNA repair gets physical: mapping an XPA-binding site on ERCC1. *DNA Repair* (Amst). 2008 May 3;7(5):819-26.

652 Sedelnikova OA, et al. Role of oxidatively induced DNA lesions in human pathogenesis. *Mutat Res*. 2010 Apr-Jun;704(1-3):152-9.

653 Okunieff P, et al. Antioxidants reduce consequences of radiation exposure. *Adv Exp Med Biol*. 2008;614:165-78.

654 Ling G. *Life at the Cell and Below Cell Level: The Hidden History of a Fundamental Revolution in Biology*. Pacific Press, NY, 2001.

655 Pollack GH. *Cells, Gels and the Engines of Life: A New Unifying Approach to Cell Function*. Ebner & Sons Publishers, Seattle, WA., 2001.

656 Gerson M. A medical application of the Ling association-induction hypothesis: the high potassium, low sodium diet of the Gerson cancer therapy. *Physiol Chem Phys*. 1978;10(5):465-8.

657 Rehydrated with low-temperature cooking, such as placing the dried seaweed into properly prepared Miso soup.

658 Cope FW. Successful therapy of heart disease by high potassium together with low sodium in accord with predictions from the associated cation, structured water concept of the cell. *Physiol Chem Phys*. 1979;11(1):93-4.

659 Phillips PA. Reduced thirst after water depravation in healthy elderly men. *NEJM*. 1984;311(12):753-9.

660 Cope FW. A medical application of the Ling association-induction hypothesis: the high potassium, low sodium diet of the Gerson cancer therapy. *Physiol Chem Phys*. 1978;10(5):465-8.

661 Gann DL, Lo S. *Double Helix Water: Has the 200-year-old mystery of homeopathy been solved?* D and Y Publishing Las Vega, NV, 2009.

662 Frankenberg-Schwager M. The role of nonhomologous DNA end joining, conservative homologous recombination, and single-strand annealing in the cell cycle-dependent repair of DNA double-strand breaks induced by H(2)O(2) in mammalian cells. *Radiat Res*. 2008 Dec;170(6):784-93.

663 Carrel A. Growth-promoting function of leucocytes. *J Exp Med*. 1922 Sep 30;36(4):385-91.

664 Alexander P, et al. Effect of nucleic acids from immune lymphocytes. *Nature*. 1967;213:569-72.

665 Kanwar JR, et al. Molecular and biotechnological advances in milk proteins in relation to human health. *Curr Protein Pept Sci*. 2009 Aug;10(4):308-38.

666 Zimecki M, Artym J. Therapeutic properties of proteins and peptides from colostrum and milk. *Postepy Hig Med Dosw* (Online). 2005;59:309-23.

667 Rusu D, Drouin R, Pouliot Y, Gauthier S, Poubelle PE. A bovine whey protein extract stimulates human neutrophils to generate bioactive IL-1Ra through a NF-kappaB- and MAPK-dependent mechanism. *J Nutr*. 2010 Feb;140(2):382-91.

668 Desmedt M, et al. Macrophages induce cellular immunity by activating Th1 cell responses and suppressing Th2 cell responses. *J Immunol*. 1998 Jun 1;160(11):5300-8.

669 Glod J, et al. Monocytes form a vascular barrier and participate in vessel repair after brain injury. *Blood*. 2006 Feb 1;107(3):940-6.

670 Murata Y, Shimamura T, Hamuro J. The polarization of Th1/Th2 balance is dependent on the intracellular thiol redox status of macrophages due to the distinctive cytokine production. *International Immunology*. 2002 Feb;14(2):201-212.

671 Glod J, et al. Monocytes form a vascular barrier and participate in vessel repair after brain injury. *Blood*. 2006 Feb 1;107(3):940-6.

672 Wilson GB, Fudenberg HH. Use of In Vitro Assay Techniques to Measure Parameters Related to Clinical Applications of Transfer Factor Therapy. USPTO 4610878, 1986 Sep 9.

673 Konishi RK, et al. Antitumor effect induced by a hot water extract of chlorella vulgaris: resistance to meth-a-tumor growth mediated by CE-induced polymorphonuclear leukocytes. *Cancer Immunol Immunother*. 1985;19:73-8.

674 Alexander P, et al. Effect of nucleic acids from immune lymphocytes. *Nature*. 1967;213:569-72.

675 Playford RJ, et al. Bovine colostrum is a health food supplement which prevents NSAID induced gut damage. *Gut*. 1999 May;44(5):653-8.

676 Leone-Bay A. Natural peptides to drugs – fourth international congress. *IDrugs*. 2010 Jun;13(6):369-71.

677Kumamoto S. Method of human cell culture. *USPTO* 4,468,460, 1984; In: Kay, R.A., Microalgae as food and supplement. *Critical Reviews in Food Science and Nutrition*. 1991;30(6):567.

678 Jensen GS, Drapeau C. The use of in situ bone marrow stem cells for the treatment of various degenerative diseases. *Medical Hypotheses*. 2002;59(4):422–428

679 Iivanainen A, Hölttä E, Ståhls A, Andersson LC. Colostral growth factors. Possible role in bovine udder epithelial cell regeneration. *Acta Vet Scand*. 1992;33(3):197-203.

680 Rudman D, et al. Effects of human growth hormone in men over 60 years old. *NEJM*. 1990; 323:1-6.

681 Starr M, *Hypothyroidism Type 2*. New Voice Publications, 2005.

682 Salomon F, et al. The effects of treatment with recombinant human growth hormone on body composition and metabolism in adults with growth hormone deficiency. *NEJM*. 1989; 321:1797-803.

683 Tamai K, et al. Role of Hrs in maturation of autophagosomes in mammalian cells. *Biochem Biophys Res Commun*. 2007; 360:721-7.

684 Casalino L, et al. Control of embryonic stem cell metastability by L-proline catabolism, *Journal of Molecular Cell Biology*. 2011 Feb 8;1–15 (Advanced online publishing).

685 Ferguson MW, O'Kane S. Scar-free healing: from embryonic mechanisms to adult therapeutic intervention. *Philos Trans R Soc Lond B Biol Sci*. 2004 May 29;359(1445):839-50.

686 Zeman K, et al. Effect of thymic extract on allogeneic MLR and mitogen-induced responses in patients with chronic active hepatitis B. *Immunological Investigations*. 1991 Dec;20(7):545.

687 Fujisawa K, et al, Therapeutic effects of liver hydrosylate preparation on chronic hepatitis-A double blind, controlled study. *Asian Med J*. 1984;26:497-526.

688 Cope FW. Pathology of structured water and associated cations in cells (the tissue damage syndrome) and its medical treatment. *Physiol Chem Phys*. 1977;9(6):547-53.

689 Cope FW. Successful therapy of heart disease by high potassium together with low sodium in accord with predictions from the associated cation, structured water concept of the cell. *Physiol Chem Phys*. 1979;11(1):93-4.

690 Cope FW. A medical application of the Ling association-induction hypothesis: the high potassium, low sodium diet of the Gerson cancer therapy. *Physiol Chem Phys*. 1978;10(5):465-8.

691 Tiwari P, Kumar A, Ali M, Mishra KP. Radioprotection of plasmid and cellular DNA and Swiss mice by silibinin. *Mutat Res*. 2010 Jan;695(1-2):55-60.

692 Bakuridze AD, et al. Radio protective drug production from fresh leaves of Aloe arborescens Mill. *Georgian Med News*. 2009 Jun;(171):80-3.

693 Lee HJ, et al. Modification of gamma-radiation response in mice by green tea polyphenols. *Phytother Res*. 2008 Oct;22(10):1380-3.

694 Vos O. Role of endogenous thiols in protection. *Adv Space Res*. 1992;12(2-3):201-7.

695 Bump EA, Brown JM. Role of glutathione in the radiation response of mammalian cells in vitro and in vivo. *Pharmacol Ther*. 1990;47(1):117-36.

696 Rotkovska D, et al. Radioprotective effects of aqueous extract from Chlorococcal freshwater algae (Chlorella kessieri) in mice and rats. *Strahlenther Onkol*. 1989;165:813.

697 Vacek A, et al. Radioprotection of hemopoiesis conferred by aqueous extract from Chlorococcal algae (Ivastimul) administered to mice before irradiation. *Exp Heamotol*. 1990;18:237-73.

698 Qishen P, et al. Radioprotective effect of extract from spirulina platensis in the mouse bone marrow cells studied by using the micronucleus test. *Toxicology Let*. 1989;48:165.

699 Ivanova KG, et al. The biliprotein C-phycocyanin modulates the early radiation response: a pilot study. *Mutat Res*. 2010 Jan;695(1-2):40-5.

700 Madhyastha HK, et al. uPA dependent and independent mechanisms of wound healing by C-phycocyanin. *J Cell Mol Med*. 2008 Dec;12(6B):2691-703.

701 Chang CJ, et al. A novel phycobiliprotein alleviates allergic airway inflammation by modulating immune responses. *Am J Respir Crit Care Med*. 2011 Jan 1;183(1):15-25.

702 Wagner R, Silverman EC. Chemical protection against X-radiation in the guinea-pig. I. Radioprotective action of RNA and ATP. *Int J Rad Biol*. 1967;12:101-12.

703 Maisin J, et al. Yeast ribonucleic acid and its nucleotides as recovery factors in rats receiving an acute whole-body dose of X-rays. *Nature*. 1960;186:487-95.

704Newman EA, et al. Effect of Nucleic Acid Supplements in the Diet on Rate of Regeneration of Liver in Rats. *Am J Physiol*. 1951;164:251.

705Dimitriadis, G.J., Introduction of Ribonucleic Acids into Cells by Means of Liposomes. *Nucleic Acid Research*. 1978;5:1381.

706 Sugahara T, et al. Effect of an alkaline-hydrolyzed product of yeast RNA on the survival of repeatedly irradiated mice. *Radiation Res*. 1966;29:516-22.

707 Ebel JP, et al. Study of the therapeutic effect on irradiated mice of substances contained in RNA preparations. *Int J Rad Biol*. 1969;16:201-9.

708 Lourau M, Lartigue O. The influence of diet on the biological effects produced by whole body irradiation. *Experientia*. 1950;6:25.

709 Bogdanov I. Observation on the therapeutic effect of the anti-cancer preparation from Lactobacillus bulgaricus (LB-51) tested on 100 oncological patients. *Laboratory for the Research and Protection of Biologically Active Substances*. Sofia, Bulgaria, 1982.

710 Simon G. Intestinal flora in health and disease. In: *Physiology of the Intestinal Tract*. Edited by L. Johnson, Raven Press, NY, NY, 1981:1361-80.

711 Chaitow L, Trenev N. *Probiotics*. Thorsons, Hammersmith, London, 1990:144.

712 Martin RA. *The Psychology of Humor: An Integrative Approach*. Elsevier Academic Press, London, UK, 2007;pp.289-90, 304, 313-31.

713 See: http://www.soundhealthoptions.com/jbab/index.html.

714 See: http://www.soundhealthoptions.com/future.html.

715 Ankri R, Lubart R, Taitelbaum H. Estimation of the optimal wavelengths for laser-induced wound healing. *Lasers Surg Med*. 2010 Oct;42(8):760-4.

716 Tennant J. *Healing is Voltage: The Key to Pain Control and Chronic Disease*. Tennant Institute for Integrative Medicine and Pain Control, Irving, TX. 972-580-1156.

717 Becker RO, et al., Iontopheretic system for stimulation of tissue healing and regeneration. *USPTO* 5,814,094, September 29, 1998.

718 Becker RO. "Process and products involving cell modification." *USPTO* 4,528,265, 1985 Jul 9.

719 Bjorn Nordenstrom. *Biologically Closed Electric Circuits: Clinical, Experimental and Theoretical Evidence for an Additional Circulatory System*. Nordic Medical Publications: Stockholm (1983). ASIN: B001P8AZ7O.

720 Rau CS, et al. Far-infrared radiation promotes angiogenesis in human microvascular endothelial cells via extracellular signal-regulated kinase activation. *Photochem Photobiol*. 2011 Mar-Apr;87(2):441-6.

721 Calabrese V, Cornelius C, Dinkova-Kostova AT, Calabrese EJ. Vitagenes, cellular stress response, and acetylcarnitine: relevance to hormesis. *Biofactors*. 2009 Mar-Apr;35(2):146-60.

722 Sgouros G, Knox SJ, Joiner MC, Morgan WF, Kassis AI. Bystander and low–dose-rate effects: are these relevant to radionuclide therapy? *J Nucl Med* 2007 Oct;48(10):1685-7.

723 Marples B, Wouters BG, Joiner MC. An association between the radiation induced arrest of G(2)-phase cells and low-dose hyper-radiosensitivity: a plausible underlying mechanism? *Radiat Res.* 2003;160:38–45.

724 Kokjima S. Induction of glutathione and activation of immune functions by low-dose, whole-body irradiation with gamma-rays. *Yakugaku Zasshi.* 2006 Oct;126(10):849-57.

725 Kojima S, Ishida H, Takahashi M, Yamaoka K. Elevation of glutathione induced by low-dose gamma rays and its involvement in increased natural killer activity. *Radiat Res.* 2002 Mar;157(3):275-80.

726 La fixité du milieu intérieur est la condition de la vie libre; Oevures xvi, 113 = Phénomènes de la vie, tome i, cited in J. M. D. Olmstead, Claude Bernard, Physiologist , Harper & Brothers, NY, 1938; p. 254.

727 Luckey TD. *Hormesis with Ionizing Radiation*. CRC Press. 1980.

728 *Hormesis: A Revolution in Biology, Toxicology and Medicine*. Edited by Mark P. Mattson and Edward J. Calabrese, Humana Press, 1st Edition, 2009 Nov 9.

729 Wing S, et al. A case control study of multiple myeloma at four nuclear facilities. *Ann Epidem*. 2000 Apr;10(3):144-53.

730 Wing S, Richardson DB, Hoffmann W. Cancer risks near nuclear racilities: the importance of research design and explicit study hypotheses. *Environ Health Perspect*. 2011 Apr;119(4):417-21.

731 Bernard C. Principes de médecine expérimentale. Ou de l'expérimentation appliquée à la physiologie, à la pathologie et à la thérapeutique (Écrits entre 1858 et 1877). Paris: Les Presses universitaires de France, 1947;pp.266-9.

732 Yamaoka K, et al. Basic study on radon effects and thermal effects on humans in radon therapy. *Physiol Chem Phys Med NMR.* 2001;33(2):133-8.

733 Nikolopoulos D, Vogiannis E, Petraki E, Zisos A, Louizi A. Investigation of the exposure to radon and progeny in the thermal spas of Loutraki (Attica-Greece): results from measurements and modeling. *Sci Total Environ*. 2010 Jan 1;408(3):495-504.

734 Vogiannis E, Nikolopoulos D. Modelling of radon concentration peaks in thermal spas: application to Polichnitos and Eftalou spas (Lesvos Island – Greece). *Sci Total Environ*. 2008 Nov 1;405(1-3):36-44.

735 Yamaoka K, et al. The elevation of p53 protein level and SOD activity in the resident blood of the Misasa radon hot spring district. *J Radiat Res* (Tokyo). 2005 Mar;46(1):21-4.

736 Florou H, et al. Field observations of the effects of protracted low levels of ionizing radiation on natural aquatic population by using a cytogenetic tool. *J Environ Radioact*. 2004;75(3):267-83.

737 Florou H, Trabidou G, Nicolaou G. An assessment of the external radiological impact in areas of Greece with elevated natural radioactivity. *J Environ Radioact*. 2007 Jan 24;93(2):74-83.

738 Yamaoka K, et al. Basic study on radon effects and thermal effects on humans in radon therapy. *Physiol Chem Phys Med NMR*. 2001;33(2):133-8.

739 Azzam EI, Raaphorst GP, Mitchel REJ. Radiation-induced adaptive response for cells. *Radiation Research*. 1994;138(1):S28-S31.

740 De Toledo SM, et al. Adaptive response to low-dose/low-dose-rate gamma rays in normal human fibroblasts: the role of growth architecture and oxidative metabolism. *Radiation Research*. 2006;166(6):849-57.

741 Yamaoka K, et al. The elevation of p53 protein level and SOD activity in the resident blood of the Misasa radon hot spring district. *J Radiat Res* (Tokyo). 2005 Mar;46(1):21-4.

742 Olsson MG, et al. Bystander cell death and stress response is inhibited by the radical scavenger α(1)-microglobulin in irradiated cell cultures. *Radiat Res*. 2010 Nov;174(5):590-600.

743 Zeman K, et al. Effect of thymic extract on allogeneic MLR and mitogen-induced responses in patients with chronic active hepatitis B. *Immunological Investigations*. 1991 Dec;20(7):545.

744 Fujisawa K, et al, Therapeutic effects of liver hydrosylate preparation on chronic hepatitis-A double blind, controlled study. *Asian Med J*. 1984;26:497-526.

745 Firat E, et al. Delayed cell death associated with mitotic catastrophe in gamma-irradiated stem-like glioma cells. *Radiat Oncol*. 2011 Jun 10;6(1):71.

746 Aypar U, Morgan WF, Baulch JE. Radiation-induced genomic instability: are epigenetic mechanisms the missing link? *Int J Radiat Biol*. 2011 Feb;87(2):179-91.

747 Koturbashi I, et al. Epigenetic dysregulation underlies radiation-induced transgenerational genome instability in vivo. *Int J Radiat Oncol Biol Phys*. 2006 Oct 1;66(2):327-30.

748 Yamaoka K, et al. Biochemical comparison between radon effects and thermal effects on humans in radon hot spring therapy. *J Radiat Res* (Tokyo). 2004 Mar;45(1):83-8.

749 See: http://doctorapsley.com/default.aspx.

750 See: http://doctorapsley.com/ACT.aspx.

751 See: http://doctorapsley.com/ICCT.aspx.

752 See: http://doctorapsley.com/FoundingFathers.aspx.

753 See: http://doctorapsley.com/ContributingFounders.aspx.

754 See: http://doctorapsley.com/FourPillars.aspx.

755 Man-made.

756 NRC: National Research Council (2005). Biologic effects of ionizing radiation VII: Health risks from exposure to low levels of ionizing radiation. *National Academy of Science*, Washington DC. See: http://www.nirs.org/press/06-30-2005/1.

757 Ling GN. *Life at the Cell and Below Cell Level: A Hidden History of a Fundamental Revolution in Biology*. Pacific Press, NY. 2001.

758 Tennant J. *Healing is Voltage: The Key to Pain Control and Chronic Disease*. Tennant Institute for Integrative Medicine and Pain Control, Irving, TX. 972-580-1156. See: http://www.tennantinstitute.com/TIIM_MAC/Welcome.html

759 The Phase Angle is the angle between resistance and impedance, and is measured in degrees. See: http://www.rjlsystems.com/bia-disease-states.shtml.

760 Polarized multi-layers of water were discovered by Gilbert Ling and Freeman Cope back in the 1970's via MRI analysis of living cells. This is the specific kind of water found in healthy cells, and forms the gel state along with select minerals and select proteins which keep the cell functioning optimally. It is water that is highly organized, molecule by molecule, and enables transfer of information and substances to proceed in ways and at speeds necessary to maintain the chemical reactions of life at normal body temperatures. See: http://www.physiologicalchemistryandphysics.com/pdf/PCP38-2_ling.pdf.

761 Graeub R. *The Petkau Effect: Nuclear Radiation, People and Trees*. Four Walls Eight Windows, NY, 1992.

762 Mangano JJ. Childhood leukemia in US may have risen due to fall out from Chernobyl. *BMJ*. 1997 Apr 19;314(7088):1200.

763 Wing S, Richardson DB, Hoffmann W. Cancer risks near nuclear facilities: the importance of research design and explicit study hypotheses. *Environ Health Perspect*. 2011 Apr;119(4):417-21.

764 Busby C, Bramhall R. Is there an excess of childhood cancer in North Wales on the Menai Strait, Gwynedd? Concerns about the accuracy of analyses carried out by the Wales Cancer Intelligence Unit and those using its data. Green Audit Aberystwyth. Occasional Paper. 2005/3, Nov 5th 2005;p. 19.

765 Yablokov AV, Nesterenko VB, Nesterenko AV. Chernobyl: Consequences of the Catastrophe for People and the Environment. *Ann N Y Acad Sci*. 2009 Dec;1181(1).

766 Yablokov AV, Nesterenko VB, Nesterenko AV. 8. Atmospheric, water, and soil contamination after Chernobyl. *Ann N Y Acad Sci*. 2009 Nov;1181(1):223-36.

767 Takada A, Song Y. Beef contamination spreads in Japan as cattle eat radiation-tainted straw. *Bloomberg,* 2011 Jul 15. See: http://www.bloomberg.com/news/2011-07-15/beef-contamination-spreads-in-japan-as-cattle-eat-radiation-tainted-straw.html.

768 See: http://www3.nhk.or.jp/daily/english/21_06.html.

769 Willacy M. Greenpeace finds radioactive sea life off Japan. Updated May 26, 2011 19:42:00. See: http://www.abc.net.au/news/2011-05-26/greenpeace-finds-radioactive-sea-life-off-japan/2732786.

770 The China Post News Staff. Nuclear fallout to bypass Taiwan en route to HK: experts. *The China Post*, Updated Wednesday, March 30, 2011 11:32 pm TWN. See: http://www.chinapost.com.tw/taiwan/national/national-news/2011/03/30/296643/Nuclear-fallout.htm.

771 Marran CL. Contamination: From Minamata to Fukushima - A slowly emerging picture. *Asian-Pacific Journal.* Japan Focus. See: http://www.japanfocus.org/-Christine-Marran/3526.

772 Nesterenko AV, Nesterenko VB, Yablokov AV. 12. Chernobyl's radioactive contamination of food and people. *Ann N Y Acad Sci.* 2009 Nov;1181(1):289-302.

773 Yablokov AV. 9. Chernobyl's radioactive impact on flora. *Ann N Y Acad Sci.* 2009 Nov;1181(1):237-54.

774 Yablokov AV. 10. Chernobyl's radioactive impact on fauna. *Ann N Y Acad Sci.* 2009 Nov;1181(1):255-80.

775 See: http://www.enviroreporter.com/2011/07/hepa-filter-july-19-2011/.

776 See Table Chart – Pastuerized, Homogenized Milk at: http://www.nuc.berkeley.edu/node/2174.

777 Diehl A. Radionuclides in drinking water: implementing the national primary drinking water regulations for radionuclides, Norm Water Paper 9-2003, 40 CFR 141, 2001 Apr 4; revised 2010 Nov 24:1-30.

778 Wing S, Richardson DB, Hoffmann W. Cancer Risks near Nuclear Facilities: The Importance of Research Design and Explicit Study Hypotheses. *Environ Health Perspect.* 2011 Apr;119(4):417-21.

779 Bouville A, et al. Radiation dosimetry for highly contaminated Belarusian, Russian and Ukrainian populations, and for less contaminated populations in Europe. *Health Phys.* 2007 Nov;93(5):487-501.

780 Nesterenko AV, Nesterenko VB, Yablokov AV. 12. Chernobyl's radioactive contamination of food and people. *Ann N Y Acad Sci.* 2009 Nov;1181:289-302.

781 Nesterenko VB, Nesterenko AV. 13. Decorporation of Chernobyl radionuclides. *Ann N Y Acad Sci.* 2009 Nov;1181:303-10.

782 Yablokov AV, Nesterenko VB, Nesterenko AV. 15. Consequences of the Chernobyl catastrophe for public health and the environment 23 years later. *Ann N Y Acad Sci.* 2009 Nov;1181:318-26.

783 Ilnytskyy Y, Kovalchuk O. Non-targeted radiation effects-An epigenetic connection. Mutat Res. 2011 Sep 1;714(1-2):113-25.

784 Aypar U, Morgan WF, Baulch JE. Radiation-induced genomic instability: are epigenetic mechanisms the missing link? *Int J Radiat Biol.* 2011 Feb;87(2):179-91.

785 Please note that the guidelines provided in my book are not intended to replace the medical advice of your doctor, or to be construed as medical advice or treatment. A qualified holistic physician familiar with radioprotective therapeutics may largely agree and order their patients to follow the guidelines presented *in Fukushima Meltdown & Modern Radiation: Protecting Ourselves and Our Future Generations.* But you should not expect all physicians to prescribe a medical treatment plan consistent with the guidelines provided in this book. Therefore, in considering and evaluating the procedures, steps, and protocols provided in *Fukushima Meltdown & Modern Radiation*, note that for the reader they are intended to exclusively serve as educational facts, guidelines, and principles known to be scientifically

consistent with successful methods in radioprotection. If you do decide to implement any of these protocols into your dietary, please first consult with a qualified holistic physician familiar with radioprotective therapeutics in order to avoid any potential adverse events which may pertain to your specific state of health. This disclaimer applies to the entire contents of this book, especially Chapter Seven and especially to all asterisks appearing in the text.

786 Gray J. *State of the Evidence: The Connection Between Breast Cancer and the Environment* (and) Nudelman J, Engle C. *From Science to Action, Breast Cancer Fund*, Sixth Edition, 2010. See: http://www.breastcancerfund.org/assets/pdfs/publications/state-of-the-evidence-2010.pdf; pp.62-3.

787 See: http://www.fpl.com/environment/nuclear/nukebook_measuring_radiation.shtml

788 AK, HI, WA, OR, CA, IA, NV, upper Mid-West and Northern Plains (North Dakota and Minnesota), PA, Mississippi and western Kentucky, plus all SE states from Missouri up to Virginia, and likely two or more NE states (NY & VT).

789 See: http://www.ncdc.noaa.gov/sotc/hazards/2011/3; http://www.ncdc.noaa.gov/sotc/hazards/2011/4 ; http://www.ncdc.noaa.gov/sotc/hazards/2011/5.

790 See: http://www.ncdp.mailman.columbia.edu/files/Nuclear_041411.pdf.

791 Circle are approximate: http://modernsurvivalblog.com/images/2011/03/united-states-nuclear-reactors-location-map-large.jpg.

792 Mangano JJ. Cancer mortality near Oak Ridge, Tennessee. *International Journal of Health Service*. 1994;24(3):521-33.

793 Gould JA. *The Enemy Within: The High Cost of Living Near Nuclear Reactors*. Four Walls Eight Windows, NY, NY, 1996;pp.39-40, 131-2.

794 Stueve D. Management of pediatric radiation dose using Philips fluoroscopy systems DoseWise: perfect image, perfect sense. *Pediatr Radiol*. 2006;36(Suppl 2):216.

795 Brown PH, et al. Optimization of a fluoroscope to reduce radiation exposure in pediatric imaging. *Pediatr Radiol*. 2000;30:229–35.

796 den Boer A, et al. Reduction of radiation exposure while maintaining high-quality fluoroscopic images during interventional cardiology using novel x-ray tube technology with extra beam filtering. *Circulation*. 1994;89:2710–14.

797 Lu ZF, et al. New automated fluoroscopic system for pediatric applications. *J Appl Clin Med Phys*. 2005;6:88–105.

798 Yablokov AV, Nesterenko VB. 1. Chernobyl contamination through time and space. *Ann N Y Acad Sci*. 2009 Nov;1181(1):5-30.

799 Yablokov AV, Nesterenko VB, Nesterenko AV.15. Consequences of the Chernobyl catastrophe for public health and the environment 23 years later. *Ann N Y Acad Sci*. 2009 Nov;1181(1):318-26.

800 Evets LV, et al. The biological effect of low-level radiation doses on the morphological composition of the peripheral blood in children. *Radiobiologiia*. 1992 Sep-Oct;32(5):627-31.

801 Yablokov AV, Nesterenko VB, Nesterenko AV.15. Consequences of the Chernobyl catastrophe for public health and the environment 23 years later. *Ann N Y Acad Sci.* 2009 Nov;1181(1):318-26.

802 Nesterenko VB, Nesterenko AV, Babenko VI, Yerkovich TV, Babenko IV. Reducing the 137Cs-load in the organism of "Chernobyl" children with apple-pectin. *Swiss Med Wkly.* 2004 Jan 10;134(1-2):24-7.

803 Nesterenko VB, Nesterenko AV. 13. Decorporation of Chernobyl radionuclides. *Ann N Y Acad Sci.* 2009 Nov;1181(1):303-10.

804 Weinberg HS, et al. Very high mutation rate in offspring of Chernobyl accident liquidators. *Proc Biol Sci.* 2001 May 22;268(1471):1001-5.

805 Taiwan lies just ~1,400 miles (2220 kilometers) from the heart of Japan, a fraction of the distance from Japan to the west coast of North America. According to EURAD simulations, Taiwan should have been inundated with radioactive fallout from the Fukushima Catastrophe. See April 6-21, especially for surface level fallout of 137Cs: http://www.woweather.com/weather/news/fukushima?LANG=us&VAR=euradsfc.

806 Marović G, Franić Z, Sencar J, Bituh T, Vugrinec O. Mosses and some mushroom species as bioindicators of radiocaesium contamination and risk assessment. *Coll Antropol.* 2008 Oct;32 Suppl 2:109-14.

807 Ould-Dada Z, et al. Radionuclides in fruit systems: model prediction-experimental data intercomparison study. *Sci Total Environ.* 2006 Aug 1;366(2-3):514-24.

808 Taira Y, et al. Current concentration of artificial radionuclides and estimated radiation doses from 137Cs around the Chernobyl Nuclear Power Plant, the Semipalatinsk Nuclear Testing Site, and in Nagasaki. *J Radiat Res* (Tokyo). 2011;52(1):88-95.

809 Dancause KN, et al. Chronic radiation exposure in the Rivne-Polissia region of Ukraine: implications for birth defects. *Am J Hum Biol.* 2010 Sep-Oct;22(5):667-74.

810 Strezov A, Nonova T. Influence of macroalgal diversity on accumulation of radionuclides and heavy metals in Bulgarian Black Sea ecosystems. *J Environ Radioact.* 2009 Feb;100(2):144-50.

811 Melintescu A, Galeriu D. Dynamic model for tritium transfer in an aquatic food chain. *Radiat Environ Biophys.* 2011 Aug;50(3):459-73.

812 Fuma S, et al. Environmental protection: researches in National Institute of Radiological Sciences. *Radiat Prot Dosimetry.* 2011;146(1-3):295-8.

813 Morita T, Fujimoto K, Kasai H, Yamada H, Nishiuchi K. Temporal variations of 90Sr and 137Cs concentrations and the 137Cs/90Sr activity ratio in marine brown algae, Undaria pinnatifida and Laminaria longissima, collected in coastal areas of Japan. *J Environ Monit.* 2010 May;12(5):1179-86.

814 Tseng CL, Weng PS, Sun KH. Sorption of low-level radwaste by Spirulina. *Radioisotopes.* 1986 Oct;35(10):540-2.

815 Horikoshi T, Nakajima A, Sakaguchi T. Uptake of uranium by various cell fractions of Chlorella regularis. *Radioisotopes.* 1979 Aug;28(8):485-8.

816 See: http://www.youtube.com/watch?v=aGonec787ME&feature=related.

817 See: http://www.youtube.com/watch?v=UKdsjyUB_dI.

818 See: http://www.youtube.com/watch?v=7Gr8hr4W64E&NR=1&feature=fvwp.

819 See multi-level 137Cs simulations (especially at ground level) for April: http://www.woweather.com/weather/news/fukushima?LANG=us&VAR=euradsfc.

820 See: http://www.helencaldicott.com/2011/04/how-nuclear-apologists-mislead-the-world-over-radiation/.

821 Yablokov AV. 11. Chernobyl's radioactive impact on microbial biota. *Ann N Y Acad Sci*. 2009 Nov;1181(1):281-4.

822 Apsley, JW. *The Regeneration Effect: Spearheading Regeneration with Wild Blue Green Algae*. Genesis Communications, LLC, Northport, AL, 1996.

823 Apsley JW. *The Regeneration Effect: A Professional Treatise on Self Healing*. Genesis Communications, LLC, Northport, AL, 1996.

824 Personal email communication, dated September 12, 2011 2:24:00 PM EDT, from Arnie Gundersen relaying a forward email from Marco Kaltofen, PE (Civil, MA) of Boston Chemical Data Corp., 2 Summer Street, Suite 14, Natick, MA USA 01760, with the following report: "The Klamath Falls air filters came in at an average of 0.15 uSv/hr, with a 0.13 uSv/hr. empty chamber level. The SD was 0.013 uSv/hr. No peaks were detected except K40."

825 Urbano G, et al. The role of phytic acid in legumes: antinutrient or beneficial function? *J Physiol Biochem*. 2000 Sep;56(3):283-94.

826 Jagtap VS, et al. An effective and better strategy for reducing body burden of radiostrontium. *J Radiol Prot*. 2003 Sep;23(3):317-26.

827 Besson B, Pourcelot L, Lucot E, Badot PM. Variations in the transfer of radiocesium (137Cs) and radiostrontium (90Sr) from milk to cheese. *J Dairy Sci*. 2009 Nov;92(11):5363-70.

828 Escartin C, et al. Nuclear factor erythroid 2-related factor 2 facilitates neuronal glutathione synthesis by upregulating neuronal excitatory amino acid transporter 3 expression. *J Neurosci.* 2011 May 18;31(20):7392-401.

829 Calabrese V, et al. Cellular stress response: a novel target for chemoprevention and nutritional neuroprotection in aging, neurodegenerative disorders and longevity. *Neurochem Res*. 2008 Dec;33(12):2444-71.

830 Illian TG, Casey JC, Bishop PA. Omega 3 Chia seed loading as a means of carbohydrate loading. *J Strength Cond Res*. 2011 Jan;25(1):61-5.

831 Jagtap VS, et al. An effective and better strategy for reducing body burden of radiostrontium. *J Radiol Prot*. 2003 Sep;23(3):317-26.

832 Besson B, Pourcelot L, Lucot E, Badot PM. Variations in the transfer of radiocesium (137Cs) and radiostrontium (90Sr) from milk to cheese. *J Dairy Sci*. 2009 Nov;92(11):5363-70.

833 Escartin C, et al. Nuclear factor erythroid 2-related factor 2 facilitates neuronal glutathione synthesis by upregulating neuronal excitatory amino acid transporter 3 expression. *J Neurosci.* 2011 May 18;31(20):7392-401.

834 Calabrese V, et al. Cellular stress response: a novel target for chemoprevention and nutritional neuroprotection in aging, neurodegenerative disorders and longevity. *Neurochem Res*. 2008 Dec;33(12):2444-71.

835 Illian TG, Casey JC, Bishop PA. Omega 3 Chia seed loading as a means of carbohydrate loading. *J Strength Cond Res*. 2011 Jan;25(1):61-5.

836 Select antioxidants found in fruits and vegetables will negate positive chelation effects of IP-6).

837 Gautam S, Platel K, Srinivasan K. Influence of combinations of promoter and inhibitor on the bioaccessibility of iron and zinc from food grains. *Int J Food Sci Nutr*. 2011 May 27.

838 Urbano G, et al. The role of phytic acid in legumes: antinutrient or beneficial function? *J Physiol Biochem*. 2000 Sep;56(3):283-94.

839 Setlow P. I will survive: DNA protection in bacterial spores. *Trends Microbiol*. 2007 Apr;15(4):172-80.

840 Nicholson WL, et al. Bacterial endospores and their significance in stress resistance. *Antonie Van Leeuwenhoek*. 2002 Aug;81(1-4):27-32.

841 Kuad P, et al. Complexation of Cs+, K+ and Na+ by norbadione A triggered by the release of a strong hydrogen bond: nature and stability of the complexes. *Phys Chem Chem Phys*. 2009 Nov 28;11(44):10299-310.

842 Korovitch A, et al. Norbadione a: kinetics and thermodynamics of cesium uptake in aqueous and alcoholic media. *J Phys Chem B*. 2010 Oct 7;114(39):12655-65.

843 Periyakaruppan A, Kumar F, Sarkar S, Sharma CS, Ramesh GT. Uranium induces oxidative stress in lung epithelial cells. *Arch Toxicol*. 2007 Jun;81(6):389-95.

844 Only take under your Doctor's orders. Folks on sodium restricted diets should ask their doctor about potassium bicarbonate solutions in place of sodium bicarbonate (baking soda).

845 Only take under your Doctor's orders. For folks with known allergy to aspirin, do not take Willow Bark or other salicylates. Stop taking immediately if it becomes difficult to breathe arises or in the event a skin rash occurs.

846 Henge-Napoli MH, et al. Efficacy of 3,4,3-LIHOPO for reducing the retention of uranium in rat after acute administration. *Int J Radiat Biol*. 1995 Oct;68(4):389-93.

847 Fatome M. [Management of accidental internal exposure]. *J Radiol.* 1994 Nov;75(11):571-5. And see: http://amarillo.com/stories/022708/bus_9691333.shtml.

848 Fukuda S, et al. The effects of bicarbonate and its combination with chelating agents used for the removal of depleted uranium in rats. *Hemoglobin*. 2008;32(1-2):191-8.

849 Maisin J, et al. Yeast ribonucleic acid and its nucleotides as recovery factors in rats receiving an acute whole-body dose of X-rays. *Nature*. 1960;186:487-95.

850 Ebel JP, et al. Study on the therapeutic effect on irradiated mice of substances contained in RNA preparations. *Int J Radiat Biol*. 1969;16:201-9.

851 Wagner R, Silverman EC. Chemical protection against X-radiation in the Guinea-Pig. I. Radioprotective action of RNA and ATP. *Int J Radiat Biol*. 1967;12:101-12.

852 Atasoy BM, et al. Prophylactic feeding with immune-enhanced diet ameliorates chemoradiation-induced gastrointestinal injury in rats. *Int J Radiat Biol*. 2010 Oct;86(10):867-79.

853 Prinz PN, et al. Higher plasma IGF-1 levels are associated with increased delta sleep in healthy older men. *J Gerontol A Biol Sci Med Sci*. 1995 Jul;50(4):M222-6.

854 Tembo AC, Parker V. Factors that impact on sleep in intensive care patients. *Intensive Crit Care Nurs*. 2009 Dec;25(6):314-22.

855 Weinhouse GL, Schwab RJ. Sleep in the critically ill patient. *Sleep*. 2006 May;29(5):707-16.

856 Irwin M, et al. Partial night sleep deprivation reduces natural killer and cellular immune responses in humans. *FASEB J*. 1996;10:643-53.

857 Stehle JH, von Gall C, Korf HW. Melatonin: a clock-output, a clock-input. *J Neuroendocrinol*. 2003 Apr;15(4):383-9.

858 Sancar A, et al. Circadian clock control of the cellular response to DNA damage. *FEBS Lett*. 2010 Jun 18;584(12):2618-25.

859 Hill SM, et al. Molecular mechanisms of melatonin anticancer effects. *Integr Cancer Ther*. 2009 Dec;8(4):337-46.

860 Carrillo-Vico A, et al. The modulatory role of melatonin on immune responsiveness. *Curr Opin Investig Drugs*. 2006;7:423-431.

861 Guerrero JM, Reiter RJ. Melatonin-immune system relationships. *Curr Top Med Chem*. 2002 Feb;2(2):167-79.

862 Hill SM, et al. Molecular mechanisms of melatonin anticancer effects. *Integr Cancer Ther*. 2009 Dec;8(4):337-46.

863 Wright CE, Erblich J, Valdimarsdottir HB, Bovbjerg DH. Poor sleep the night before an experimental stressor predicts reduced NK cell mobilization and slowed recovery in healthy women. *Brain Behav Immun*. 2007;21:358-63.

864 Patt BT. Prevalence of obstructive sleep apnea in patients with chronic wounds. *J Clin Sleep Med*. 2010 Dec 15;6(6):541-4.

865 Meier-Ewert HK, et al. Effect of sleep loss on C-reactive protein, an inflammatory marker of cardiovascular risk. *J Am Coll Cardiol*. 2004;43:678-83.

866 Irwin MR, Carrillo C and Olmstead R. Sleep loss activates cellular markers of inflammation: sex differences. *Brain Behav Immun*. 2010;24:54-7.

867 Moldofsky H. Central nervous system and peripheral immune functions and the sleep-wake system. *J Psychiatry Neurosci*. 1994;19:368-74.

868 See: http://en.wikipedia.org/wiki/Music_therapy.

869 See: http://www.soundhealthinc.com/pdf/mac_degen.pdf.

870 Nelson A, et al. The impact of music on hypermetabolism in critical illness. *Curr Opin Clin Nutr Metab Care*. 2008 Nov;11(6):790-4.

871 Lysenko IuN, Niko'lskiĭ ID. Achieving the optimal functional status of the body through the use of suggestion, music and bioacoustic means. *Gig Sanit.* 1989 Nov;(11):86-7.

872 Konstantinov KV. Restoration of interhemispheric symmetry of the bioelectrical brain activity in patients with neurasthenic syndrome by bioacoustic correction. *Biull Eksp Biol Med.* 2000 Feb;129(2):139-41.

873 See: http://2011tappingworldsummit.com/2011_free_event_access.html.

874 Shaharudin SH, et al. The use of complementary and alternative medicine among Malay breast cancer survivors. *Altern Ther Health Med.* 2011 Jan-Feb;17(1):50-6.

875 Epel F, et al. Can meditation slow rate of cellular aging? Cognitive stress, mindfulness, and telomeres. *Ann N Y Acad Sci.* 2009 Aug;1172:34-53.

876 See: http://www.krill-oil-benefits.com/phospholipids.php.

877 Caldicott H. Medical and economic costs of nuclear power. Online Opinion. 2009 Sep 14; see: http://www.onlineopinion.com.au/view.asp?article=9422&page=2.

878 See: http://www.nuclearfreeplanet.org/articles/you-can-stop-the-expansion-of-australias-biggest-uranium-mine-.html.

879 Fernandes A. Uranium mining 'a health risk.' Science Alert, *ScienceNetwork WA*, 2009 Aug 18; see: http://www.sciencealert.com.au/news/20091808-19572.html.

Index

29718783R00164

Made in the USA
Lexington, KY
05 February 2014